IMMUNITY

DON'T BUY IT, BUILD IT

ANJALI (HOLISTIC NUTRITIONIST AND LIFESTYLE COACH)

ISBN 979-888530742-0

Contents

For the people who want to build their immunity and have long-term health goals.

A Brief Note To The Readers

In covid 19 pandemic, I lost so many people from my family. I have seen the fear and pain of losing someone. There was a time when my whole family got tested covid positive, I can't forget that time. My parents were infected.

The initial 4-5 days were a bit critical because they had a fever of about 103-104F, low oxygen levels, weakness...., I observed so many things during that phase. They didn't take a single pill.

Our focus was on a balanced diet, quality sleep, and other aspects like I blocked the way of negativity(no social media and phone calls), daily early morning sunlight, emotional detox through meditation, family time (we spent so much quality time with each other). After 25 days they were back to normal life.

I learned one thing very strongly, "don't panic". It's just a phase and it will pass. You need to be mindful rather than being tense and panicked, I'm saying this because I have seen this.

My patients, known ones, sent me so many links of superfoods with one common question, will this product boost my immunity?

Through all these queries, I found there is no lack of knowledge about immunity boosters because you just need to type "how to boost immunity"? And so many drinks and "nuskhe" will appear on your screen. But most people don't know that it's not only about eating things, but immunity is way more than this, you need to work on all the aspects.

Everyone is unique, and I strongly believe that no one can understand you more than yourself. My goal is to make things easy for you so that you can apply them and for that, I have put things clear and simple.

In this book, I have tried to put all the necessary things that can help you in the journey to understand the core of immunity and how you can work on it. Through this book, I want to share the knowledge that I have gathered in the past few years. I kept the scientific ideas as clear as possible and understandable through diagrams, flow charts for the general readers

Acknowledgment

I want to thank my supreme guide and teacher the Godfather **"Shiv baba"** who has enlightened my path at every footstep in life by the dint of his Godly Wisdom. By whose grace I am in a position to furnish every task smoothly and peacefully.

I'm grateful to my mother for her support during this amazing journey of book writing. After my mother, the major credit goes to my friend Abhishek Goklani, who believed in me when I was struggling to believe in myself.

"Perfection is endless"- this thing can stop you from initiating something.
-Anjali

CHAPTER I

UNDERSTANDING THE WORLD OF MICROBES AND THE IMMUNE SYSTEM

Described by the US National Library of Medicine as "the most complex system that the body has", our immune system is a vast constellation of cells and molecules spanning every nook and cranny of our bodies.

We fear of bacterias, germs that they will infect us but let me clear this up, microbes(bacterias) live on us, in us, and around us. With every breath you take, you inhale thousands of bacteria, and with every bite you eat, you can ingest a million more. The bugs comprising our microbiota are actually our biggest health allies. And 99 percent of them won't hurt us.

Our lifelong task of trying to balance our immunity means relying heavily on certain exposures to good germs for proper calibration. Why?

Well, when we look through evolution, our immunity developed through times of great peril, interacting with germs of all kinds-good and bad.

When operating optimally, this immune-microbial alliance creates a dialogue that underpins our immunity, selecting, activating, and terminating many of its various components as we need them, helping us distinguish how susceptible we are to infection and our likelihood of getting an autoimmune disease. This dialogue even controls how our brains function.

There are four different immune systems in the body. Each of these systems operates separately, but all follow the same owner's manual and communicate with each other. The largest one is found in the gut(gastrointestinal tract), where 70 to 85% of our immunity resides.

There is another immune system in the liver called the kupffer cells. The third comprises the white blood cells found in the bloodstream. Finally, the most potent immune system in the body is in the brain and is made of glial cells.

Does aging affect immunity?

As we get older, though, our immune function declines. Is this just an inevitable consequence of aging? Or could it be because dietary quality also tends to go down in older populations? To test the theory that inadequate nutrition could help explain the loss in immune function as you age, researchers split eighty-three volunteers between sixty-five and eighty-five years old into two groups.

The control group ate fewer than three daily servings of fruits and vegetables, while the experimental group consumed at least five servings a day. They were all then vaccinated against pneumonia, a practice recommended for all adults over the age of sixty-five.

The goal of vaccination is to prime your immune system to produce antibodies against a specific pneumonia pathogen should you ever become exposed. Compared with the control group, this was after only a few months of eating just a few extra servings of fruits and vegetables a day. That is how much control the fork may exert over immune function.

Certain fruits and vegetables may give the immune function an extra boost.

Why do we get sick, if we have a defense system (immune

system)?

When harmful pathogens attack our body, most of the time our bodies win the fight against germs, but sometimes they lose. People who 'never get sick' may catch a slight cold now and again or suffer an occasional ache and pain. This makes sense when you realize that we live in a microbial world, and the microbes were here first.

There are up to 1 trillion microbial species on Earth, and only a minute fraction of them cause disease. So vilifying all microbes for the sake of a few is a mistake, and possibly one of our biggest(you'll discover why in chapter 4).

Let's look at how the infection spreads. Take rhinovirus, the cause of the common cold, for instance. Roughly one in five people carry the rhinovirus at any given time in the tissues of their nasal passages(the prefix 'rhin' in Greek literally means 'the nose'). To infect you, these germs need three things:

*A way to get out of the reservoir(the person sitting near who is sick).

*A mode of transportation to a new home(that person sneezing- a sneeze produces 40,000 droplets and you can get infected by inhaling just one)

*A way to get into their new home(you)

Another classic route for the spread of germs is poor hygiene, especially inadequate hand washing.

Let's bust a myth-

You must have heard this in childhood 'Put on a jacket or you'll catch a cold'. But it's now dismissed as an age-old misconception because it's the "virus", not the "temperature".

It has been shown that when you are exposed to the cold for a prolonged time you may not be able to launch the most robust immune attack. While this effect might be marginal in most healthy people, older people, young kids, or those with underlying health issues may have an even harder time fighting off the virus.

So, best heed your parents' advice and bundle up when heading out in the cold. Wearing a scarf in winter does warm the air in the back of your throat, making it less hospitable for those seasonal viruses that prefer cool air.

Do vaccines always work?

Research shows that 85-95 percent are effective for most infections. But as we know we all are so different. And so are disease-causing germs. So the effectiveness of each vaccine differs. Even our unique microbiota (you will see this in chapter 4) can impact your response to vaccines. Flu is particularly tricky.

The vaccine's effectiveness depends on the strains the public-health agencies pick- and sometimes they get it wrong. The 2018 vaccine was only 23 percent effective at preventing flu.

CHAPTER II

INTRODUCTION TO THE IMMUNE SYSTEM

The term "immune system" is derived from the Latin word immunis, meaning untaxed or untouched, which is fitting, given that the immune system protects the body from foreign invaders. It is our foundation for wellbeing. When it comes to maintaining good health, the immune system is our most precious asset.

The immune system is composed of various organs, white blood cells(leukocytes), and proteins called antibodies that form alliances against trespassing pathogens threatening the body, the immune system.

The immune system also includes lymphatic organs(such as lymph nodes, bone marrow, and spleen), apart from the nervous system, which is the most complex organ system humans possess. Our immune system is essential for survival. It protects us from pathogens. Without an immune system, your body would be open to attack from bacteria, viruses, parasites, fungi. It looks out your body against the invaders.

When harmful microbes enter the body, the body produces white blood cells to fight the infection. White blood cells identify the harmful microbes, produce antibodies to fight them, and help other immune responses to occur.

The interesting thing about them is **"they remember the attack"**.

The bone marrow is our immune cell factory where new immune cells are born from stem cells-a blank canvas cell with the capacity to evolve into any one of our numerous immune cell types.

Do we really need to "boost" our immunity?

NO, we need a balanced immunity because of the way your immune system is designed to work, you definitely wouldn't want it to be boosted. An underactive or overactive immune system causes health issues.

The immune system is like a series of switches-a rheostat requiring constant tweaking to get it just right. Attempting to 'boost' the cells of the immune system is complicated. There are so many different kinds that respond to so many different microbes in so many ways. Which should you boost? And how much? So far, there is no clear and single answer.

The best way to strengthen your immune system is through a combined approach that you will read in the following chapters.

MAJOR ORGANS OF THE IMMUNE SYSTEM

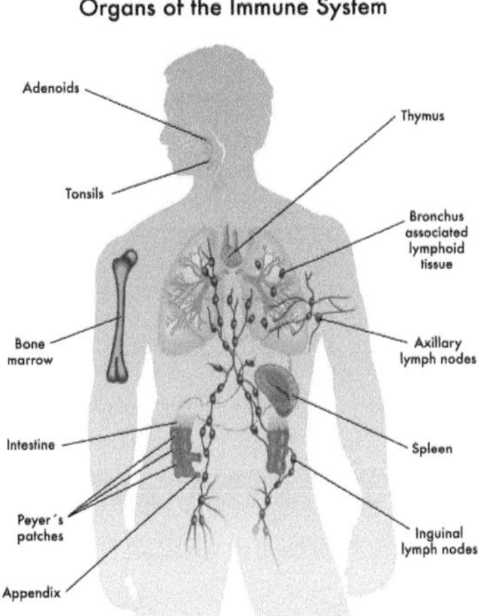

1. **Thymus**- the thymus is an organ located in the upper chest. Immature lymphocytes leave the bone marrow and fight their way to the thymus where they are "educated" to become mature T-lymphocytes.

2. **Liver**- the liver is the major organ responsible for synthesizing proteins of the complement system. In addition, it contains a large number of phagocytic cells that ingest bacteria in the blood as it passes through the liver.

3. **Bone marrow**- the bone marrow is the location where all the cells of the immune system begin their development from primitive stem cells.

4. **Tonsils**- tonsils are a collection of lymphocytes in the throat.

5. **Lymph nodes**- lymph nodes are a collection of B- lymphocytes and T-lymphocytes throughout the body. Cells congregate in lymph

nodes to communicate with each other.

6. **Spleen**- the spleen is a collection of T-lymphocytes, B-lymphocytes, and monocytes. It serves to filter the blood and provides a site for organisms and cells of the immune system to interact.

7. **Blood**- blood is the circulatory system that carries cells and proteins of the immune system from one part of the body to another.

SOME IMPORTANT CELLS INVOLVED IN THE IMMUNE SYSTEM

1. **B-cells**- these lymphocytes arise in the bone marrow and differentiate into plasma cells which in turn produce immunoglobulins(antibodies)

2. **Cytotoxic T cells**- these lymphocytes mature in the thymus and are responsible for killing infected cells.

3. **Helper T- cells**- these specialized lymphocytes "help" other T-cells and B-cells to perform their functions.

4. **Plasma cells**- these cells develop from B-cells and are the cells that make immunoglobulins for the serum and the secretions.

5. **Immunoglobulins**- these highly specialized protein molecules, also known as antibodies, fit foreign antigens, such as polio, like a lock and key. Their variety is so extensive that they can be produced to match all possible microorganisms in our environment.

6. **Neutrophils**- a type of cell found in the bloodstream that rapidly ingests microorganisms and kills them.

7. **Monocytes**- these are the type of phagocytic cell found in the bloodstream that develops into a macrophage when it migrates to tissues.

8. **Red blood cells**- the cells in the bloodstream which carry oxygen from the lungs to the tissues.

9. **Dendritic cells**- they are the antigen-presenting cells of the immune system. Their function is to process the antigen material and present it on the cell surface to the T cells of the immune system. They act as messengers between the innate and adaptive immune systems.

10. **Natural killer cells-type of lymphocytes and a component of the innate immune system.** They play a major role in the host rejection of both tumors and virally infected cells. Natural killer(NK) cells recognize changes in our own cells. These cells are crucial to our health, rapidly responding to kill our own cells when they get infected with a virus.

They are the body's main cancer surveillance tool. With specialized receptors, they patrol the body inspecting each cell. They respond to newly formed tumors and abnormal growth of cells.

Types of immunity-

1. INNATE IMMUNITY

We are born with this immunity, it is present by birth in our body(first line of defense against invaders). Innate immunity is vital for life, but it only has a short-term memory. The innate immune response is fast-acting and non-specific, which means it does not respond differently based on the specific virus or bacteria which it detects.

The innate immune system encompasses physical barriers, chemical, and cellular defenses.

1. **Physical barrier** protects the body from invasion. These include things like the skin and eyelashes.

2. **Chemical barriers** are defense mechanisms that can destroy the harmful agent. Examples include tears, mucus, and stomach acid.

3. **Cellular defenses** of the innate immune responses are non-specific. These cellular defenses identify pathogens and substances that are potentially dangerous and take steps to neutralize or destroy them.

2.**Adaptive(acquired)immunity-**

This immunity develops throughout our lives. We develop adaptive immunity when we're exposed to diseases or get vaccinated. The adaptive immune system is like a library of memory cells, unlike the innate immune system.

Information on every virus, bacteria, or fungi that ever invaded your body and was defeated by your immunity is achieved by this immune system, identifying them by their molecular shape. This is called immunological memory. Adaptive immunity is controlled by the lymphocytes(a type of leukocytes/white blood cells) known as B lymphocytes and T lymphocytes.

T lymphocytes are the master controllers, sent out into the body, controlling the levels of many other arms of immunity. They recognize, respond to and remember "antigen".

B lymphocytes are special reconnaissance unit-the antibody producers. Each B cell makes one type of antibody that's specific for one foreign molecular signature.

They produce antibodies-protein(gamma globulin) that recognizes foreign substances(antigen)and attach themselves to them. B-lymphocytes are powerless to penetrate the cell so the job of attacking these target cells is left to T lymphocytes.

Each of us has a repertoire of T and B lymphocytes, adding a layer of individual exclusivity to our immunity and, consequently, our health. An immune system that doesn't produce a huge variety of unique T and B lymphocytes will probably miss or "not see" certain germs or viruses, and these could go on, unchallenged, to cause disease. This happens during aging.

3. PASSIVE IMMUNITY

This type of immunity is "borrowed" from another source, but it does not last indefinitely. For instance,a baby receives antibodies from the mother through the placenta before birth and breast milk following birth. This passive immunity protects the baby from some infections during the early years of their life.

How does immune response coordination happen?

All of the immune cells work together, so they need to communicate with each other. They do this by secreting increased levels of a special protein molecule called "cytokines". The term "cytokine" is derived from a combination of two Greek words "cyto" meaning cell and "kinos" meaning movement.

Cytokines are cell signaling molecules that aid cell to cell communication in immune responses and stimulate the movement of cells toward sites of inflammation, infection, and trauma. Examples of cytokines include the agents interleukin and interferon which are involved in regulating the immune system's response to inflammation and infection.

Functions of the immune system(brief)-

THE MAIN TASKS OF THE BODY'S IMMUNE SYSTEM ARE-

a. To fight disease-causing germs(pathogens)like bacteria, viruses, fungi, or parasites and remove them from the body.

b. To recognize and neutralize harmful substances from the environment.

c. To fight disease-causing changes in the body, such as cancer cells.

CHAPTER III

FOUR PILLARS OF IMMUNITY

Embarked on detox week after binge eating over the weekend, but forgot to slot in the exercise in your daily routine? Started your day with an intense workout or yoga, but ended it with an entire pizza? Doing all things right, but failing to get enough sleep.

If this is your pattern or you can relate to this then it's time to realize that; like how Rome wasn't built in a day, good health can't be obtained in a short period. It's a long-term commitment.

The immune system is precisely that- a system, not a single entity. To function well, it requires balance and harmony.

We come back to basics repeatedly. Everything is not complex in life, let's keep this simple - nutrition, exercise, sleep, mindfulness. Sounds very basic and easy but it's the foundation of good health.

PILLAR -1

NUTRITION-

"Tell me what you eat, and I will tell you what you are."

(Jean Anthelme Brillat- Savarin, $18^{th}/19^{th}$- century French lawyer, politician, and epicure)

Our immune system consists of organs, tissues, and millions of cells throughout the body that, together, create a protective network. These cells rely on a healthy diet for proper functioning. Lack of proper nutrition has been linked to decreased immunity and increased risk of illness.

Our immune system not only depends on macronutrients such as protein, carbohydrate, and fat to build antibodies, we also need micronutrients, vitamins, minerals, antioxidants. This diverse collection of nutrients helps the body to identify invaders, break them down and dispose of them.

However, with our hectic, grab-and-go lifestyles, we know it can be hard to get all the nutrients we need from our diet alone, which is why taking a supplement may be a good option.

Before we start this, let's be clear: there is no such thing as an immunity diet. If someone says this particular diet can "boost" your immunity, they are probably fooling you.

If something that can really help you then it's only balanced nutrition, it plays a crucial role in building one's immunity. I cant pen down all the things here but will go through the few essential and useful pointers for strong immunity.

a) Antiviral foods- some foods and herbs like oregano, sage, tulsi, fennel, peppermint, licorice, garlic, turmeric, coconut oil, star anise, ginger slows down the growth of the virus and helps in fighting against the infection.

GINSENG is a Chinese-origin herb, it is a well-known immune modulator, especially roots. Roots(mostly), stems, leaves of ginseng, and their extracts have been used for maintaining immune homeostasis and enhancing resistance to illness or microbial attacks.

b)Vitamin D- An adequate amount of vitamin d is essential for immunity and to decrease inflammation in the body. People who have low vitamin D levels have shown higher susceptibility to upper respiratory tract infections. The natural source of vitamin D is sunshine, sit in early morning sunlight(7 AM to 9 AM) for 30 minutes. Wear light and minimum clothes during sunbathing. If you are taking vitamin d supplements, don't forget vitamin k2 because vitamin d works well only if you have vitamin k2, approximately half of which is produced by our microbiome(gut bugs).

c)Vitamin A- it is a micronutrient that is crucial for maintaining vision, promoting growth and development. Vitamin A is known as anti-inflammatory because of its critical role in enhancing immune function, it is involved in the development of the immune system and plays regulatory roles in cellular immune response and humoral immune process.

It helps regulate the immune system and protects from infections by keeping skin and tissues in the mouth, stomach, intestines, and respiratory system healthy. Vitamin A is the key for the immune system to remain tolerant and anti-inflammatory, particularly in the gut.

Vitamin A from plant-based sources is called carotenoids, and from animal sources, it's called retinol. Retinol is more bioavailable than the plant source since the body has to convert carotenoids to retinol. You can get this immune nourishing vitamin from carrots, spinach, kale, sweet potatoes, red peppers, eggs, apricots, squash.

d)Vitamin C- It is a powerful antioxidant that helps in optimizing immunity as it is also known to support the development of WBC's. The best source of vitamin c is amla in any form(raw, candy, pickle), citrus fruit, guava, sauerkraut, etc.

Vitamin C appears to have even stronger effects on people who are under intense physical stress. If you do catch a seasonal lurgy, vitamin C supplement of 1-2g per day has several benefits, including reducing the symptoms and severity, decreasing recovery time by 8 percent in adults and 14 percent in children, on average.

e) Zinc- it is well known to play a central role in the immune system, zinc-deficient persons experience increased susceptibility to a variety of pathogens. Zinc works on multiple factors, from the barrier of the skin to gene regulation within lymphocytes. It is critical for the normal development and function of cells that mediate both innate and adaptive immunity.

Because zinc is not stored in the body, regular dietary intake of the mineral is important to maintain the integrity of the immune system. Zinc deficiency can lead to severe immune dysfunctions mainly affecting T helper cells, hyperammonemia(excess of ammonia in the blood).

Zinc deficiency adversely affects the growth and function of T and B cells. Recommended dietary allowances(RDA) of zinc is 10-12mg/day. The richest and good sources of zinc are pumpkin seeds, almonds, hemp seeds, legumes like chickpeas, lentils, and beans, sesame seeds, and dark chocolate.

f)Selenium- it is an essential micronutrient with antioxidant properties, it helps in lowering the oxidative stress in the body which reduces inflammation and enhances immunity.

It is important for human health in various aspects like proper thyroid hormone metabolism, cardiovascular health, prevention of neurodegeneration, and optimal immune responses.

One of the excellent sources of selenium is brazil nuts(consume 2 soaked brazil nuts in a day). Good sources of selenium are mushrooms, bananas, sunflower seeds, spinach, and legumes.

g)Probiotics and prebiotics- Both are very important for good gut health. Probiotics are living microorganisms(fermented foods, curd, rice kanji, beetroot kanji, carrot kanji, sauerkraut, kimchi, kombucha, Indian pickles, apple cider vinegar) and prebiotics is a dietary fiber that feeds friendly bacteria in the gut(apple. Banana, flaxseeds, psyllium husk, oats, onion, garlic, pear).

h)Hydration- 3 to 3.5 liters of water per day is important to detox naturally. When you drink an adequate amount of water your body's natural mechanism flush out toxins and pathogens that can cause illness. Include more liquids in your diet like tulsi concoction, soups, turmeric tea, neem giloy juice, drumstick soup.

i)Phytonutrients- phytonutrients are biologically active chemical compounds found in plants. They protect plants from pollution, viruses, pests, and bacteria. So, it's no surprise that regular consumption of phytonutrients helps prevent us from getting sick. They are the key to unlocking our own internal antioxidants that protect our delicate cellular machinery, reduce the burden of oxidative stress.

Regular consumption of phytonutrients from plant-based foods reduces the risk of infections and certain illnesses, such as cardiovascular disease and some cancers.

There are 25,000 different phytonutrients recorded across many foods. Some of the most common phytonutrients are-

1. Carotenoids- beneficial for eye health and immune system. Perhaps the best-known is lycopene(in tomatoes), which has long been associated with anti-cancer properties. While all tomatoes contain lycopene, the skin has the highest concentration and cooking is the best way to convert the lycopene into an absorbable form.

Lycopene is fat-soluble, so if you cook tomatoes with a little olive oil, the amount absorbed goes up threefold. The San Marzano heirloom variety, from southern Italy, has one of the highest levels. Found in red, dark green, and orange plants such as tomatoes, carrots, sweet potatoes, watermelon, leafy greens.

2. Flavonoids- these phytochemicals contribute to healthy cell communication. This can trigger detoxification, decrease inflammation, and reduce the risk of tumors spreading. There are many subgroups of flavonoids, such as anthocyanins and quercetin found in soybeans, onions, apples, tea, and coffee. Anthocyanins are great pain relievers with anti-inflammatory properties.

3. Resveratol- is found predominantly in grapes. Resveratrol is associated with the increased cerebral flow. It is produced by plants as a natural fungicide, found in grape skin(specifically), red wine, and berries.

4. Carnosol- a bioactive compound extracted from Mediterranean herbs such as rosemary and sage, has been found to have promising anti-cancer and anti-inflammatory properties.

5.Epigallocatechin-3-gallate(EGCG) is an immune nourishing polyphenol with natural anti- inflammatory and antioxidant properties found in quantities 16 times higher in green tea than black tea.

6. Glucosinolates- they are known for helping to regulate inflammation, metabolic functions, and stress responses. Found in cruciferous vegetables predominantly like broccoli, bok choy, Brussel sprouts, cabbage.

PILLAR-2

EXERCISE-

Our bodies were designed to move. Modern life may not allow us to stay active all day, but even a little bit of exercise can go a long way in optimizing our immunity. Engaging in 30 to 60 minutes of daily, moderate exercise can improve your body's immune response

.

Research suggests that exercise can protect your immune system from certain illnesses by flushing out bacteria from your lungs and airways, improving circulations, causing mild fluctuations in body temperature to fight infection, and releasing stress-reducing endorphins.

Exercise reduces stress hormone; cortisol and stimulates the release of serotonin and endorphins (happy hormones). It's important to understand that when you start something, continuity is a must. When you exercise you are cleaning your body by removing toxins from the body.

During exercise your blood circulation improves, your sweat production increases, water intake increases, kidneys naturally flush out toxins when you drink more water. Your body has a natural mechanism of removing toxins from the body.

No doubt proper and healthy detox diets help you in detoxification but your body's detox mechanism is much stronger than any detox diet or drink, but nowadays our lifestyle has changed whether it's about food or a sedentary lifestyle.

We want everything complex, if we get fat we'll hop on quick solutions like fat cutter drinks, pills, varieties of teas, etc. but here we need to understand one thing that we need to work on core. According to a study, after every 30 minutes, you should take a movement break. Sitting for a long period is a risk factor for early death.

There are actually four types of exercises, each one has different benefits-

#Flexibility- stretching helps to maintain flexibility, if you'll see kids they are so flexible but aging leads to loss of flexibility in muscles and tendons. Muscles shorten and don't function properly. That increases the risk for muscle cramps and pain, muscle damage, strains, joint pain and it also makes it tough to get through daily activities, such as bending down to tie your shoelaces.

While stretching the muscles routinely makes them longer and flexible, which increases your range of motion and reduces pain and risk of injury. Here are some ways to your flexibility:

Stretching various parts of the body.

Doing yoga

Static stretches

#Balance exercises- Improving your balance makes you feel steadier on your feet and helps prevent falls. It's especially important in older age when the systems that help us maintain balance- our vision, our inner ear, and our leg muscles and joints tend to break down. Here are some good balance exercises-

Heel to toe walking

Standing on one foot

Practicing tai chi poses

Walking on an uneven surface

#Endurance(aerobic)- this exercise increases your breathing and heart rate and is the main component of overall fitness programs. They keep the circulatory system lungs healthy, can stave off diabetes and heart disease, and help you build up endurance.

Some common aerobic exercises include-

Brisk walking

Jogging

Climbing the stairs

Dancing

Swimming laps

Doing yard work like raking, digging, and gardening.

#Strength exercises - It strengthens muscles, stimulates bone growth, lowers blood glucose level, assists with weight control, improves balance and posture, reduces stress and pain in the lower back and joints.

Regular strength training will help you feel more confident and capable of daily tasks like carrying groceries, gardening, and lifting heavier objects around the house.

Some examples of strength training include:

Lifting free weights

Using resistance machines at the gym

Using resistance bands to leverage your own body weight in building strength.

PILLAR-3

SLEEP-

"The shorter you sleep, the shorter your life."
Matthew Walker, Professor of Neuroscience and Psychology, University of California, Berkeley and author of '**Why we sleep.**'

We spend one-third of our lives sleeping, sleep is as essential as food and water to survive.

When we sleep our body repairs cells, restores energy, and good quality sleep reduces inflammation in the body. The study has shown that people who slept well at night before vaccination got less or no side effects like fever, headache in comparison to those who cut back on sleep.

Our white blood cells can more efficiently fight invading bacteria or viruses during sleep and if we cut down on our sleep our white blood cells get reduced.

Now how will you get to know that you slept well?

If you wake up fresh the next morning with no pains in heels, no swelling on your face, fresh mind are few signs of good quality sleep. During sleep our body detoxifies the system. That's why the first urine is a bit hot and yellowish, the crust gets deposited in the corners of the eye, and a foul smell in the mouth.

During sleep, our muscle activity slows down and we breathe slowly, now the energy that was working on the functioning of muscle activity and other works on the immune system.

Some good signs of getting enough sleep would be waking up without an alarm clock, not needing caffeine to keep you going, and being alert throughout the day.

The definition of good sleep is being asleep for more than 85 percent of the time you're in bed, waking up no more than once per night, and for fewer than 20 minutes. So if you are in bed for 10 hours, 8.5 of them should be spent sleeping.

STAGES OF SLEEP-

Yes, sleep is made up of stages, collectively known as sleep architecture. The stages comprise two types of sleep:

1. Non-rapid eye movement(NREM), also known as quiet sleep.
2. Rapid eye movement, also known as active sleep or paradoxical sleep.

The four stages of sleep-

1. NREM stage 1- light sleep- your eyes are closed, but it's easy to wake you up.

2. NREM stage 2- as your body is getting ready for deep sleep, you become less aware of your surroundings, your body temperature drops, your eye movement stops, your breathing and heart rate drop. This stage takes up about 50 percent of your time across the night.

3. NREM stage 3- known as slow-wave sleep, this is when you are deeply asleep. This is a period of deep sleep where any noises or activity in the environment may fail to wake a sleeping person. Most deep sleep tends to happen early in the first half of the night, which is why going to bed early can be helpful.

4. REM sleep- this is when you dream, usually 90 minutes after you fall asleep. While your brain is aroused with mental activities during REM SLEEP, the fourth sleep stage, your voluntary muscles become immobilized.

It's in this stage that your brain's activity most closely resembles its activity during waking hours. However, your body is temporarily paralyzed- a good thing, as it prevents you from acting out your dreams.

Babies can spend up to 50 percent of their sleep in the REM stage, compared with only about 20 percent for adults. During the deep stages of NREM sleep, the body repairs and regrows. This is our immunity fortification phase in preparation for the challenges of each day.

What does the body do when we sleep?

a)Our glymphatic system(waste clearance system) clears waste from the central nervous system(CNS) and it mostly happens during sleep.

b)During sleep, the body produces cytokines (proteins) that fight inflammation and infection.

c)Liver makes bile and other chemicals for the next day.

d)Neurons or nerve cells reorganize.

e)When we sleep brain activity increases in the areas which regulate emotions.

How can we get good sleep?

a. Don't drink tea, coffee after 5 PM. It can disturb sleep.

b. Keep your gadgets(cell phone, iPad, tablets, laptop)away before 1 hour of sleeping, gadgets emit blue light that delays melatonin(sleep-inducing hormone) production.

Do deep breathing for few minutes-

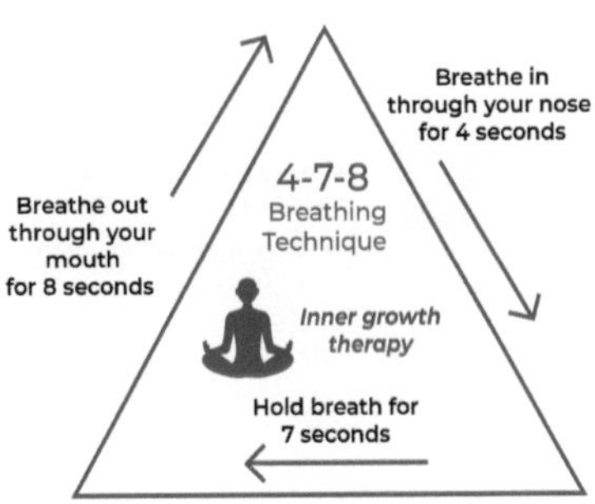

1) 4-7-8 breathing technique

2) left nostril breathing technique- in yogic terminology it is known as Chandra bhedana pranayama, Chandra bhedi pranayama. The word "Chandra" stands for the moon, while "bhedana" stands for piercing.

We have two nostrils for breathing, in yogic terms, these two nostrils are called Nadi, the right nostril is known as Surya Nadi, and the left nostril is known as Chandra Nadi.

Moon is the symbol of coolness, so by doing this pranayama we feel some coolness in our body. We sleep better in cool temperatures(not cold).

Doing this pranayama before sleeping can help you to sleep better as it helps reduce heat in the body.

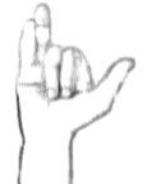

Step : 1 Make the hand form (finger Pranayama)

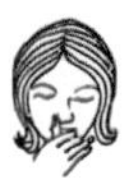

Step : 2 Close right nostril, and breathe in the left nostril.

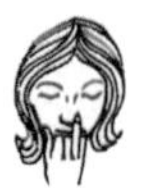

Step : 3 Close left nostril, and breathe out the right nostril.

(Repeat, alternative nostrils)

d)Write down your tasks on a notepad for the next day, it frees your mind and gives clarity to the brain.

e)Keep your diet healthy, balanced and avoid late-night dinners.

f)Exercise daily as it improves your sleep quality.

CIRCADIAN IMMUNITY

Recent studies have shown the critical role of circadian rhythm and sleep in immune system homeostasis.

What is circadian rhythm?

Circadian rhythms are daily variations in behavior and biological activity that stem from an intrinsic ability of organisms to align themselves with the environmental 24-hour light/dark cycle.

These rhythms originate from an internal biological clock that drives many aspects of human physiology, including the sleep-wake cycle and daily variations in blood pressure, body temperature, and cortisol.

Our body's daily circadian rhythm has affected our well-being in all kinds of ways. The night is biologically designated sleep time. Rhythmic circadian genetic switches are present in the majority of our immune cells.

We humans have adapted to sleep during darkness and are at our most active during daylight.

Alterations to our sleep/wake cycle affect the number of circulating master controller T cells, antibodies, and even those virus-fighting, cancer-seeking NK cells, as well as sending inflammation haywire. When our immunity is challenged during circadian disruption we see impaired immune function and unchecked inflammation.

Jet Lag causes more than just a feeling of being discombobulated-it makes you more susceptible to getting sick. In fact, even a single shift in our circadian rhythm, without sleep loss, can put us in a worse position when it comes to health.

Shift workers are more likely to suffer from fatigue, sleep deprivation, and sleeping disorders like insomnia or sleep apnoea, as well as other health problems particularly metabolic syndrome and heart disease. In 2007, the World health organization classified night-shift work as a probable carcinogen due to circadian rhythm disruption.

PILLAR-4

MINDFULNESS AND STRESS

Be mindful of stress, it can suppress the immune system's ability to break down invading pathogens.

In today's world, we are running and doing things without being mindful of our intrinsic world. We are eating food while watching television, or phones, gulping water instead of drinking. These habits may look small but these habits are like havoc for our system.

We need to be mindful of our thoughts, "negative thoughts" imbalances cortisol levels. If you think that thought is just about your inner world, you are wrong because you are emitting negativity like your phones emit blue light(that decreases melatonin hormone production).

During the covid-19 pandemic, we have learned whatever the situation is, do not be "stressed out" because it increases the severity of the disease while taming the stress reduces inflammation markers and improves the activity in the brain responsible for coordinating with an immune system.

STRESS AND IMMUNITY

The term 'stress', as it is used, was coined by Hans Selye, a pioneering Hungarian endocrinologist; he defined stress as 'the non-specific response of the body to any demand for a change.'

We only have one biological stress response, but an almost infinite number of causes(stressors). You can experience stress from your environment, your body, and your thoughts. If we define stress as anything that alters our homeostasis, for good or bad, then stress, in its many forms, is normal and vital for a healthy life.

So while stress mostly gets a bad reputation, it's not all negative. 'Stress' is a best an ambiguous term. For some, it means excitement and challenge(good stress); for many others, it reflects an undesirable state of chronic fatigue, worry, frustration, and inability to cope(bad stress).

For the latter, I prefer the term 'stressed out', which conveys the chronic nature of a negative state. In essence, stress can be normal and appropriate when it's acute'(short-lived).

Stress can be positive, keeping us alert, motivated, and ready to avoid danger. If we didn't have some stress in our lives, we would never grow as people, develop resilience and push ourselves.

The so-called 'good stress', what scientists refer to as 'eustress', is what we experience when we feel excited. Also called 'fight-or-flight' response, it's a special branch of our body's autonomic nervous system-the unconscious control center that has a built-in stress-response unit known as the sympathetic nervous system, initiating physiological changes to allow the body to combat stressful situations.

Once the stressor has been dealt with, our parasympathetic nervous system(often referred to as the 'rest-and-digest') works in concert with the sympathetic branch to gently guide us back to baseline, our pre-stress healthy and happy set point.

Our central stress-response machinery includes the hypothalamic-pituitary adrenal(HPA) axis and the sympathetic nervous system(SNS).

Basically, it's an eloquent and dynamic intertwining of the brain and body that uses hormones, neurotransmitters, and immunity molecules. It's controlled by the teeny tiny almond-sized hypothalamus in the brain, which can't tell the difference between a little stress and full overwhelm.

All it knows is that it's getting a clear neural signal from the amygdala-the brain's alarm system communicating threats and strong emotions. Upon detection of danger, this involuntary(autonomic) network releases epinephrine(most often known as adrenaline-think adrenaline rush), which creates a kind of high, giddy, heart-pumping feeling, overcoming fatigue.

The body is prepared for fight or flight within seconds. In this time, immunity is also on red alert as we get a rush of inflammatory chemicals into the blood.

Now inflammation is pretty important for defense, but it's also damaging and requires policing. Almost simultaneously, there is the release of cortisol, a type of steroid hormone known as a glucocorticoid.

This is the next critical step in the stress response, allowing us to survive moments of panic, as cortisol helps the body maintain essential functions, like blood flow, so we don't faint in pressurized situations. Collectively, this rush of stress also inhibits the action of the rational thinking brain, forcing us to fixate on the threat in hand.

HOW CAN WE MANAGE STRESS?

1. Deep breathing- when we breathe it sends a signal to the brain to calm and relax, it enables more air to flow in your body and relaxes nerves. Do pranayama, kapalbhati, bhramari on an everyday basis.

2. Exercise- when we exercise our body releases happy hormones that lower stress automatically.

3. Balanced diet- include more varieties of fruits and vegetables, add whole grains to your diet.

4. Meditation- when you meditate the adrenal gland produces less cortisol, your body uses oxygen more efficiently, your brain gets more clear, and creativity increases. It helps to achieve emotional stability.

5. Write it- it seems basic but it works wonders when you write it gives more clarity to our thoughts. If you write down your tasks before sleeping it also helps you to sleep with a relieved mind.

6. Socialise- spending time with family, friends, and kids help release a hormone called oxytocin, a natural stress reliever.

7. Self-talk - we forget this precious thing, it's the most important thing. Take out time for yourself, you should know what's going on in your inner world because ultimately that will define your reaction to the outer world.

8. Affirmations- yes, Do you know about the subconscious mind? All your habits of thinking and acting are stored in the subconscious mind. If you give some positive affirmations to the subconscious mind for 21 days, it memorizes it and works according to that.

Some positive affirmations-

1. My body is healthy and disease-free.
2. I'm a positive soul.
3. I'm stress-free.
4. I'm a happy and vibrant soul.
5. I radiate happiness and peace.

9. Laughter- stimulates blood circulation in the heart, lungs, and muscles. Laughter releases neuropeptide that helps fight stress and potentially more serious illnesses,

It relieves pain by causing the body to produce its own natural painkillers. One minute of anger weakens your immune system for 4 to 5 hours, one minute of laughter boosts the immune system for up to 24 hours.

WHEREVER YOU ARE, BE THERE TOTALLY(mindfulness)
-Eckhart Tolle

CHAPTER IV

GUT HEALTH ROLE IN IMMUNITY

"We are not individuals. We are ecosystems with microbial partners that are involved in the development(particularly in early life)and function of essentially every organ, including immunity."
(Graham Rook, Emeritus Professor of Medical Microbiology, University College London)

Based on current estimates, every one of us is home to a community of 38 trillion microbes(microbiome)- accounting for half of each of us(by cell count). Yes, the trillions of bacterias(microbiome/ microbiota) that are majorly housed in your gut are responsible for 70% to 85% of your immune system.

The microbiome contains 99% non-pathogenic and 1% pathogenic microbes.

Microbes exist everywhere on and in the human body. They are clustered around the barriers of our bodies(skin, urinary tract, lungs, gut), reinforcing these boundaries, the good bacterias out-competing the bad bacterias: on the skin, bacteria promote healing; in the vagina they guard against unwanted yeast; and in mouth, they break down the food and protect teeth and gums.

No single part of our body is sterile, with microbes making up to 2kg of our body weight. The essential task of the gut immune system is to maintain a balance between immune reaction and tolerance.

The foundation of good gut health begins with what and how you eat. Other than our diets microbiome also gets negatively affected by our oversantised environments, increased antibiotic use, and modern-day lifestyle.

It's not just antibiotics, there are other commonly used prescribed drugs- including metformin, proton pump inflammatory drugs(NSAIDs)- that have recently been associated with changes in the gut microbiome composition.

How to minimize antibiotic dysbiosis?

Firstly, never self prescribe any antibiotic and other microbiome-influencing drugs, take these drugs only when your doctor prescribes them.

If you are on antibiotics, take the probiotics before, during, and after the course so that they can replenish gut flora.

Consume fiber-rich foods but go slow because it's an adjustment period for the body, including plenty of liquids.

THE IMMUNE SYSTEM, WHICH IS PRIMARILY IN THE GUT, IS INFLUENCED AND TAUGHT BY THE GUT MICROBIOME.
-Dr.HANAWAY

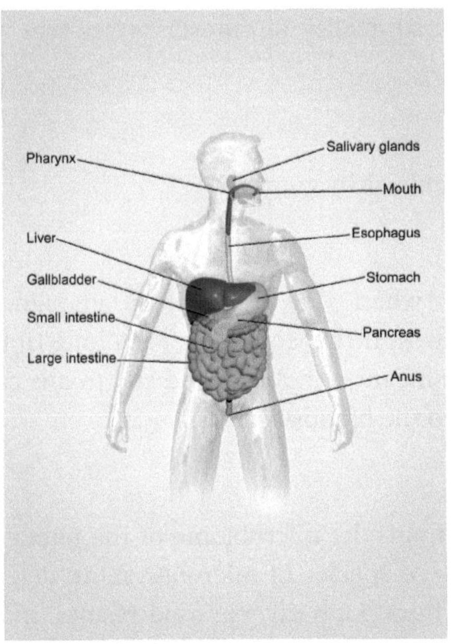

WHAT IS GUT?

The gut includes every organ involved in digesting the food, processing, and eliminating the waste from the body.

How does our gut health get compromised?

Your gut works hard to absorb the nutrients while keeping out undigested food, bacteria, and potentially harmful things that we've swallowed. At up to 40 square meters, it forms the body's largest interface with the outside world.

Modernization in the food industry changed our diet dramatically.

The food that we get in packets is processed, high in sugar, low fiber, high and bad quality fat, preservatives that have altered the gut bacteria.

Reason for the unhealthy gut-

1. Poor sleep- when you don't sleep enough, cortisol(stress hormone)increases. If this continues for a long time it can cause a leaky gut which means now your food and toxins can pass through the intestine into the bloodstream.

2. Less diverse food- the microbiome of the human body contains 300 -1000 types of species of microbes, more diverse food means more good gut flora. Less diverse food results in loss of gut flora diversity and causes inflammation in the body, poor learning, and memory, mood swings.

3. Habit of drinking too much alcohol- excess alcohol causes dysbiosis, inflammation in the body.

4. Antibiotics- antibiotics help fight bacterial infections, but they also negatively impact your immune system. Antibiotics change your microbiome, they not only kill "bad" bacteria but also kill "good" bacteria.

5. Steroids-during covid 19 pandemic many people heard about this disease called mucormycosis(black fungus)infection that usually infects people with an impaired immune system.

The use of drugs that suppress the immune system like corticosteroids(lab-made steroids that quickly fights inflammation in the body) steroid can lead to impaired immune function.(reference- BBC NEWS article)

6. Stress- it reduces gut-friendly bacteria and also reduces blood flow. When we take too much stress our cortisol levels increase and that can cause inflammation in the gut.

7. Physical activity- if you want a healthy microbiome, you need to move more, when you exercise the beneficial bacteria increases.

DID YOU KNOW?

Your gut is your second brain. Also called enteric nervous system(ENS).

CAN GUT BACTERIAS MAKE YOU SMART?

YES, research shows that gut and brain are connected, a partnership called gut-brain axis. Have you ever felt “gut-feeling” and “butterflies” in your stomach when nervous or anxious? Well then you might be getting the signal from your gut (second brain).

Fun fact- Researchers(Joslin diabetes center and Harvard Medical School) have identified a bacteria called Veillonella in the gut microbiomes of marathon runners- but not sedentary people that can boost exercise capacity. The researchers found the Veillonella bacteria preferentially metabolize lactate, which muscles produce during hard exercise, and convert it into short-chain fatty acid (SCFA)propionate which the body can then utilize to improve exercise performance.

According to John Cryan(professor of anatomy and neuroscience at the university college cork), the bacterial microbiota helps in normal brain development.

DO YOU KNOW?

The human gut is lined with 500 million neurons connected to the brain through nerves in the nervous system. The nerve that connects the central nervous system and enteric nervous system is the vagus nerve(longest nerve of the body).

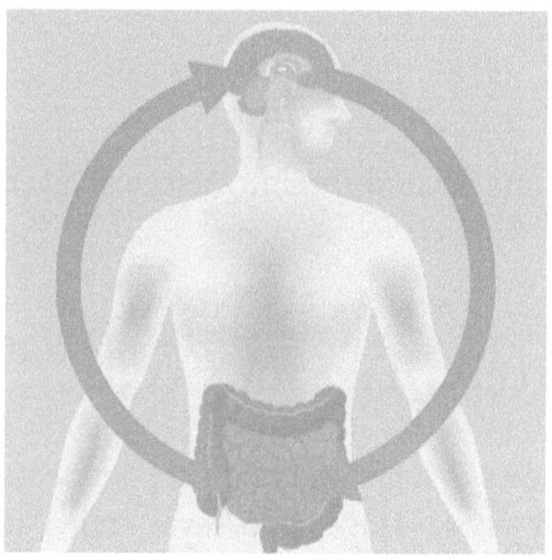

The communication between your gut and brain is called the gut-brain axis.

The gut-brain axis also communicates via chemicals like neurotransmitters, hormones.

According to MENTAL HEALTH AMERICA, “there is a strong relationship between having mental health problems and having gastrointestinal symptoms like heartburn, regurgitation, indigestion, bloating, pain, constipation or diarrhea.”

Did you know?

Researchers agree that a person’s unique microbiome is created within the first 1000 days of life, but there are things that you can do to alter your gut environment throughout your life.

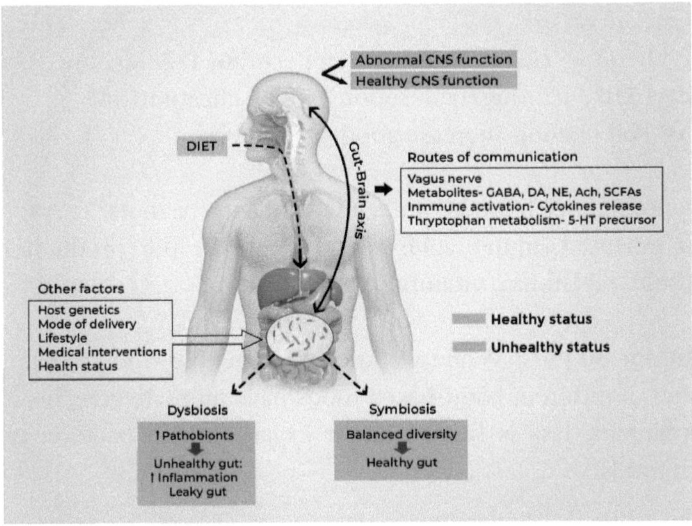

Impact of diet on the microbiome and routes of communication involved in the gut brain-axis.

Now, you must be thinking about how we can improve this gut-brain axis connection.

Some foods that are beneficial for the gut-brain axis:-

1.Fermented foods - yogurt, curd, sauerkraut,kimchi,kanjis,fermented black tea.

2. Mediterranean diet- this diet is high in fruits, vegetables, legumes, nuts, grains.

3. Fiber-rich foods- whole grains, fruits instead of juices, prebiotics.

4. Omega 3s - flaxseeds, chia seeds, walnuts, fatty fish(salmon, tuna, sardines, mackerel).

5.Polyphenol rich foods- peppermint(427mg/ounce),cocoa powder(516 mg/tablespoon), chestnut(347 mg/ ounce).Polyphenols increase good gut bacteria.

6. Tryptophan-rich foods- milk, chicken, oats, peanuts. Tryptophan is an essential amino acid, plays a role in the production of serotonin, melatonin, vitamin b3,b6.

7. Aim for 30 plus- While we know that people who eat a greater number of different plant-based foods have more diverse, healthier microbiomes, less is known about exactly which bacteria prefer which foods.

It’s particularly important to get fiber into kids when they start eating solid food to ensure that you are cultivating a diverse gut ecosystem right from the beginning.

Info fact-

It is not “curd or yogurt” it’s “curd and yogurt”, yes both dairy products are prepared differently. Curd is obtained by the process called curdling by adding rennet while the yogurt is obtained by bacterial fermentation of milk.

The conclusion of this whole information about the gut-brain axis is that you can improve your brain health by altering the microbiome.

Anything that affects the gut will always affect the brain.
Dr. Charles Majors

CHAPTER V

HEALTHY LIFESTYLE GUIDELINES

How often do you notice a wall clock that ticks away? It is something we take for granted until of course, it malfunctions and stops working properly, we do this same thing with our body, we become aware of it when it gets sick(I read these lines somewhere in a book and it blew my mind)because it is so on point, and in my practice, I see this almost daily.

You know our body is capable of self-healing, the only thing that we need to know is don't panic because only then you can make the right decision about what to do about your disease. A simple example is a headache, we pop a pill if we have a headache without thinking about why it is happening.

It could be because of a gastric problem, acid reflux, or cervical pain. That pill can suppress your symptoms but will not cure your root cause, and when you do this for the long term it becomes a disease.

If you think you'll get cured only by popping a pill then think again.

Nothing can heal you better than your own body. Let's take this example: when we get a fracture doctor puts plaster only (does not contain any healing substance), then what heals your bones is "the body" only. If it can fix your bones then why can't other ailments?

When we get a fever our body raises its temperature to fight any virus or bacteria, but we take medicine to bring down the temperature(fever), as a result, infection multiplies, and then we need antibiotics.

DO YOU KNOW?

Antibiotics put a negative impact on the gut microbiome by reducing the diversity of microbes.

"Taking an antibiotic is like dropping a bomb on your microbiome"

(Dr. Tom O'Bryan) YOU CAN FIX YOUR BRAIN

Many people recovered by covid 19 at home with proper nutrition, kadhas, and rest, another example of self-healing of the body.

In the covid-19 pandemic "how to boost immunity" was in the top search on google. You cannot boost immunity instantly by eating some superfoods or supplements. You can gain it gradually.

"Nothing is bad until and unless you make it bad by practicing it the wrong way and overdoing it."

Your body tells you everything, if something is wrong inside, the body shows symptoms outside.

One thing that I want to highlight is it's not important that if something is suiting others(neighbors, friends, family), it will suit you too. Listen and understand your body, don't follow anybody blindly.

I often hear things like "I lost weight in one month by drinking so and so concoction, you should also try this."And then we start following it religiously without knowing if it is good for you or not and when it negatively impacts your body, you blame that concoction.

"Food Is Fuel Of The Body, Every Time You Eat Is An Opportunity To Nourish The Body"

If you want to heal your body, then first you need to shift your consciousness from listening to the outer world to listen to your body.

All creatures were designed differently with different food patterns. With time only human food patterns changed because the food industry introduced a new way to eat food that is processed, high in saturated fats and this list can go on.

But have you ever seen a dog or cat eating spicy curry or anything that is not meant for their species NO because they know what food to eat. Now I'm talking about those dogs and cats who don't live inside with humans because the inside ones become like us.

We humans eat anything that looks delicious or tastes good to our taste buds.

ARE WE EATING ACCORDING TO THE FOOD INDUSTRY?

If you think you are eating according to your choice, you t might be wrong because someone else is deciding what you should like to eat or what you want to eat and that is the food industry. Yes, you heard it right.

This is something that needs your attention, if you're thinking that you are eating the sugar only when you're, making tea, lemonade, or any other sweet dish then you are probably wrong because you're eating more sugar in hidden form than the actual sugar that's because it is added in so many foods and beverages. Yes, the food industry adds sugar in maximum products to make them appealing and to increase their sales.

Why does the food industry add sugar to so many foods?

a)to preserve food, like sauces, chocolates, juices
b)to improve their texture, flavor, color
c)for fermentation
d)to provide bulk in foods

Have you ever noticed the arrangement of food products in the superstore, all the sugary and attractive packaging food arranged in the front row so your kids make you purchase it and once you'll purchase it you become the regular consumer of that product.

Why I'm telling you all this, well I want you to understand that to make your body healthy, you must surround yourself with what you want, not the food industry.

HACKS FOR SMART EATING:-

#PLAN YOUR GROCERY FOR WHOLE WEAK :

Shop vegetables from local vendors for 2-4 days so that you can get them fresh. Otherwise, when you purchase it for a whole week they do not remain that fresh, when you purchase vegetables from a superstore they might not be that fresh but they seem fresh to you because of less temperature or cold storage. Local vendors don't have any facilities like superstore so you'll get the real fresh vegetables.

Write down the stuff that you'll need for 1-week meals like pulses, legumes, snacking options like makhana, roasted chana, puffed rice, etc. When you plan the weekly food items, add nutritious options of snacking for your kids or stuff to make them at home. The problem occurs when you don't have options in healthy food then you'll choose unhealthily. When you plan your meal you're eliminating temptations almost entirely. Surround yourself with healthy foods.

TIP-1

Never go grocery shopping when you're hungry, you'll pick unnecessary unhealthy food items and more items than you need. When you're hungry it's hard to resist those attractive processed and sugary foods, so whenever you go grocery shopping make sure that you're full and also avoid going during evening snack time.

TIP-2

If you are purchasing something which is packaged like dark chocolates, cacao powder or anything make sure that you read the nutrition label, you should know what you are eating and how much preservative, trans fat, bleaching agent, monosodium glutamate(MSG), sodium phosphate, sodium nitrate, sodium nitrites, high fructose corn syrup it contains. It may take 1-2 minutes to do this but it will bring a big change in your life, mindfulness starts from small things but if you do those small ones you make it a habit(a good habit)

“Failing To Plan Is Planning To Fail”

#Switch To Homemade Drinks From Canned

In summers we want something that gives cooling effects and gives refreshment to our body but instead of choosing aerated drinks, canned juices, colored drinks you can have homemade drinks like sattu drink, wood apple juice(trust me it’s so good and cooling, it is one of my favorites), lemonade, you can also have shakes like mango shake, chikoo shake(it’s just unmatchable, must try).

These drinks are designed in such a way that they will be so palatable to your taste buds but they are nothing but sugar only, when you drink them you’ll feel satiated for some time because of sugar, as it spikes blood glucose level, dopamine(the feel-good hormone) gets released in the brain and that’s why you think that drink makes you happy, insulin gets released in large amount to drop blood glucose level.

Now what happens is the body gets confused by the wrong signal, when sugar level drops rapidly then you crave for something else. This becomes a cycle, you just crave for that particular feeling that you felt last time after consuming the particular products. Here, the only one who is actually happy is the food industry because of their increased sales and your body is a sufferer, but you have a choice to break this cycle.

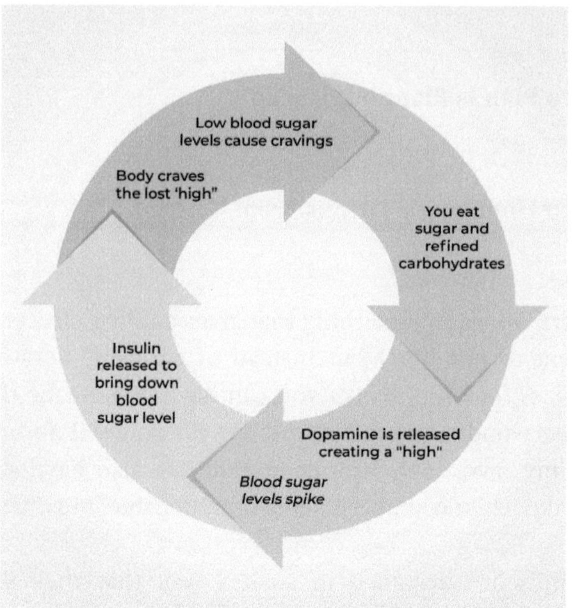

#Make Your Food Interesting

If you think a healthy diet is boring, tasteless, and bland, this hack will change your mindset. You must have heard this "I want to be healthy or to lose weight but I can't eat tasteless food".It's the most important part of eating that whatever you're eating you must feel good about, now by saying this I don't mean go eat a pizza and feel good NO, I mean to make your food tasty you have so many options because if you're not loving your food, then it's a short term thing and diet can't be a short term plan.

India is very well known for its spices, the only thing we need is to use them in the correct form and correct way. Let's take the simple example of gravy that is the base of most curry, I'm sharing my way to make gravy:

Mustard oil/ grated coconut
Cumin
Asafoetida
Tomato, green chili puree
Turmeric powder
Sea salt or rock salt
Coriander seed powder(rarely in a powdered form otherwise I like it in form of fresh leaves)

These ingredients seem less but when you try them once you'll feel the flavor of real food, usually what mistakes we do is we put so many powdered spices and then the taste of vegetable or main ingredients fades, instead of using powdered spices try to add them in fresh form.

DO YOU KNOW?

The most popular spice of the world is cumin and the most commonly used herb is coriander (cilantro).

Other spices and flavors that you can add to your food to make them tasty:

a)black pepper
b)nutmeg (crushed)
c)oregano
d)onion
e)garlic
f)basil,thyme

g)cinnamon(SriLankan rolled)
h)fenugreek
i)clove
j)rosemary
k)lemon(this can be a game-changer in food)

TIP-

Don't add any spice, salt, lemon to your salad when you're having with a meal because this increases your salt and spice consumption. If you are eating salad as a meal then you can add dressing(any spice, salt, or homemade dressing)

#Use The Technique That Mothers Use For Their Kids

You must have done this with your kid. When your kids don't like any particular vegetables what do you do? Add those vegetables in such a way that they'll not appear on the plate and the dish you prepared will also be palatable to them. Use this for yourself too, if you don't like any particular vegetable then you can blend that and knead with the flour to make chapatis, this will not only add flavor to your meal but will also add fiber, nutrients, and colors(good for gut health). Smoothies are another option to use the blender more smartly, you can make a smoothie with very basic ingredients, you will need-

a)**liquid**- coconut water/coconut milk/almond milk/oats milk/soy milk/cashew milk/cucumber/watermelon/plain water.

b)**base**-any fruit or vegetable of your choice like sapodilla, banana, papaya, apple, beetroot, carrot, orange family, mango, pomegranate, kale.

c)**sweetener**- if you add any fruit that is already sweet, you don't need to add any sweetener, but if you want to add, you can use dates, maple syrup, and honey.

d)**flavor**- sometimes we need a twist, for that you can some flavors like cacao powder, cardamom, SriLankan rolled cinnamon, mint, holy basil, coriander leaves.

Eating the same thing daily is boring and non-sustainable for the long term, trying new flavors, new fruits, and vegetables gives happiness to your body.

TIP-

If you like any particular flavor or any food try to find the healthier substitute for that or if you don't find it then create it in your kitchen, it's like therapy. In our childhood, we use to mix two different watercolors to see that which color will come, just like that try and experiment with new dishes in a healthier way for your kids too.

#Hydrate Your Body With Flavors And Quality Water

Drink water to keep your skin healthy and hydrated, to flush out those toxins from your body. We often hear this but to make it more interesting you can add detox water or infused water or in simple words water with flavor and extra health benefits. What is detox or infused water? The water infused with fresh fruits, vegetables, and herbs is called detox water. Detox water has very few calories and can be a good substitute for soda, sugary, aerated drinks. When you drink infused water it gives you refreshment and also increases your water intake.

How to make infused water, well you can make it according to your choice or you can try the following recipes(in1 liter water)-

1. add 15-20 fresh mint leaves and zucchini slices
2. lemon zest and 2-3lemon slices
3. orange slices and orange peel
4. add 10-15 basil leaves
5. fennel seeds(1 tablespoon) and green cardamom(5-6)
6. cinnamon stick (1)
7. apple slices(green or Washington)
8. curry leaves (15-20)
9. bay leaf(2-3)
10. 10. carrots and lime
11. 11. rose petals (20)
12. 12. strawberry and basil seeds(1 teaspoon)

Our body depends on water to survive. Every cell needs water to work properly, in fact, water makes 50% to 70% of body weight. Water is something that you're made of, just drinking water is not enough. Drinking quality water is the key to a healthy life.

Check these parameters in your water-

1. Total dissolved solids(TDS) should be between 50-300
2. The pH of the water should be 6.5 to 8.5
3. The hardness of water- water with less than 60ppm can be considered as soft, water with 60-120ppm moderately hard, and water with greater than 120ppm hard.

Have you ever heard these drinking water Kangen water, Evian water, black water? These all are alkaline water and loaded with natural minerals. According to report*food.ndtv.com,* Virat Kohli(INDIA captain of a cricket team)only consumes bottled water named Evian, which costs him Rs.600 per liter.

DO YOU KNOW?

Consuming RO(reverse osmosis)water for even a few months can create serious side effect-WHO.

And it has been scientifically confirmed now that drinkingn RO water causes more bodily harm and faster than most contaminants found in tap water.RO system off course removes water impurities but also removes 92-99% of beneficial calcium and magnesium.

TIP-

You can make alkaline water in your kitchen. Add 4 pieces of cucumber and 2 pieces of lemon in 1-liter water.

#CHEW YOUR FOOD

Animals feed themselves:

Men eat: but only wise men "know the art of eating".

(Jean Anthelme Brillat- Savarin)

We know that we should chew our food 32 times but how many of us do? Chewing your food properly not only eases the further process of digestion but reduces your overall food intake and prevents you from overeating. When food is not digested properly, you can suffer from indigestion, bloating, acidity, regurgitation, heartburn, constipation, headache. When we chew our food properly our nutrient absorption increases in comparison to when we just swallow food.

Tips to chew food properly-

1. Take small bites
2. Don't drink water between and just after the meal.
3. Eat food in silence and enjoy the flavors of it.
4. Stop only when the mouthful is total liquid.

#ART OF DRINKING WATER

If you drink water while standing, you don't get the required nutrition and the worst part is it does not quench your thirst. Not only this, if you don't drink water in the right way it can harm your health.

Why you don't get the benefit of drinking water while standing? When you drink this way, the water passes through the system with a straight gush, it does not reach the organs of your body to do their job. Water detoxes the body naturally but drinking it in the wrong way does the opposite as the impurities get deposited in the kidneys and bladder. It causes joint pain, bone degeneration.

Don't count only how many liters you have drank but also make sure that you drink it the right way. Sit down comfortably and then drink water, do not gulp it, sip it. When you drink this way the water passes through the designed passage and reaches every organ, brain, and boosts its activity.

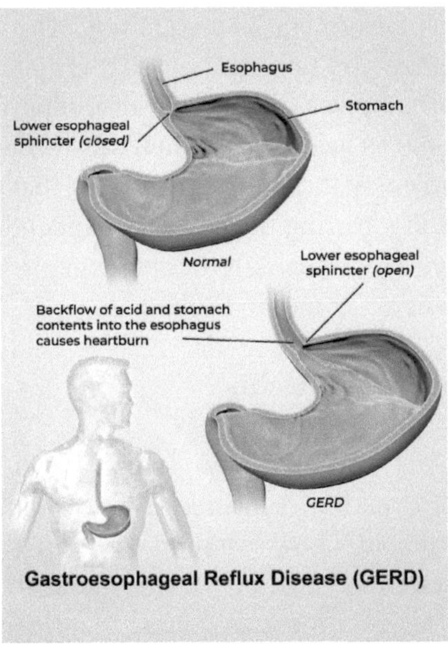

In the above picture, the lower esophageal sphincter is open, which will cause gastroesophageal reflux disease. When you drink water fastly and in a standing position, you let it flow to your gut while splashing the wall of your stomach. This gives shock to your stomach and causes long-term damage to the stomach and gastrointestinal tract.

Can Water Create Tension In Your Nerves?

When we drink water in a standing position a “fight or flight” system is activated which causes nerve tension in the body. But when you drink in a sitting position “rest and digest system"(parasympathetic system)comes into the fray, this helps in calming your senses and eases the process of digestion.

I gained with my experience that when you take care of someone, it automatically comes to you in a good way. The same thing goes with our body when you take care of what is good for it and what is not, in response, it gives you good health, superbrain, maximum energy. If your body is healthy only then this world is good for you, only then you can enjoy the luxury, the money that you have earned throughout your life. During the covid 19 pandemics, many people started their lives more healthily because they realized that your body is master when it comes to healing.

Few Steps Towards Your Health-

#Sunbath- doesn't matter how much high-end vitamin-d supplement you're taking. Sunshine is the ultimate and natural source of vitamin d. Low vitamin-d means low immunity. Deficiency of vitamin-d causes problems like high blood pressure, autoimmune diseases, muscle aches, depression, and sleep disturbances.

There is one disease called a seasonal affective disorder, it is a psychological condition that results in depression normally caused due to seasonal change. People typically experience this in winters when sunlight is less. This disease is more common in Canada and Alaska than in sunnier Florida. Studies show that depression cases increase during the wintertime due to a decrease in sunlight. Sunlight sets people's circadian rhythm by regulating the levels of melatonin and serotonin.

Types of vitamin D-

Ergocalciferol(vitamin d2)- found in plants like mushrooms, and yeasts.

Cholecalciferol(vitamin d3)- found in animals like fatty fish, and egg yolks.

VitaminD3 is more effective than vitaminD2. Cholecalciferol is produced by the body when the skin is exposed to sunlight.

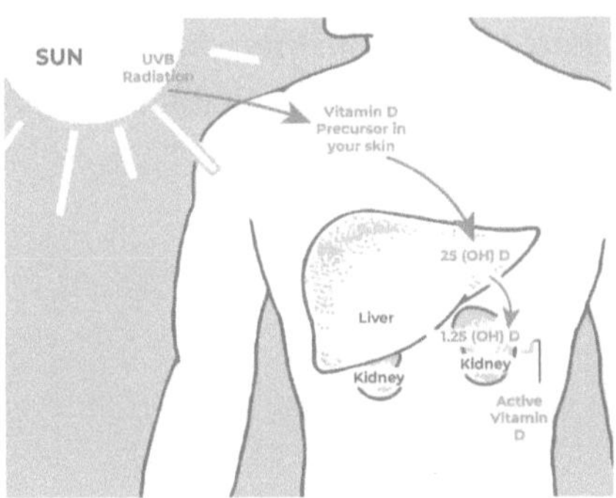

How to get vitamin D from the sun?

You can get sunshine benefits only when it reaches your skin. Wear light and minimum clothes, no sunscreen during sunbath, sit in direct sunlight(no windows), smog between the sun rays and the skin prevents absorption. Stay in sunlight for 30 min. Vitamin D is a hormone. You can never get the excess vitamin from the sun; toxicity. It's only possible when you're taking it in the form of a supplement.

How do you get to know about vitamin D levels in the body? You can know your vitamin D levels through a blood test. If you live in an area where sunlight is not proper, then you can take supplements under the guidance of your doctor. It plays a crucial role in your body so you should get it checked regularly.

#Start with alkaline foods- your body's pH is 7.35-7.45, which means your body is alkaline. When we consume acidic food our body needs to neutralize it to maintain our body's pH levels. This is done by breaking down the bones and teeth for calcium and magnesium and the muscles for ammonia to neutralize the acid. Fruits are the most alkaline foods-even citrus fruits. Give your morning kick start with alkaline foods like fruits, soaked nuts(overnight). When you eat an alkaline diet you improve your health.

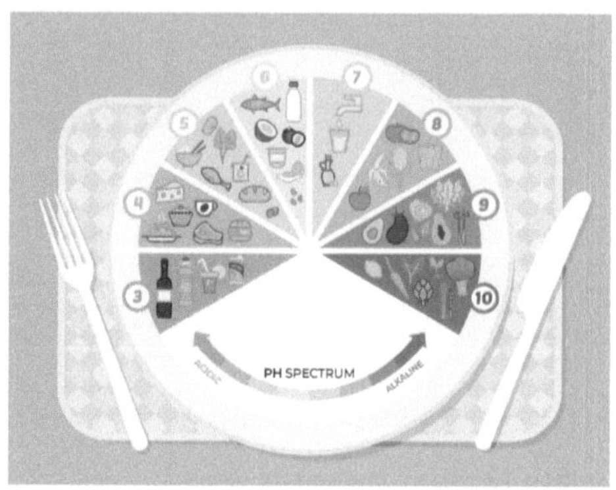

ALKALINE FOOD-

1.Fruits- banana,papaya,avocado,lemon,blueberries,fresh coconut,wood apple etc.

2.Vegetables- ash gourd(highly alkaline),beetroot,carrot,garden cress,lettuce,pumpkin,brussels sprouts,spinach,sweet potato,celery,eggplant,moringa leaves,drumstick etc.

3.Sprouts- Brussels sprouts, alfalfa sprouts, fenugreek sprouts, mung bean sprouts, amaranth sprouts, Kamut sprouts.

4.Aloe vera

5.Indian Gooseberry

6.Quinoa

ACIDIC FOODS-

1. Dairy products
2. Meat
3. Poultry
4. Eggs
5. Fish
6. Soda
7. Alcohol
8. Processed and packaged foods

Have you ever thought that why we need acidic beverages like tea, coffee, aerated beverages like colas and sodas, wines and other alcohols with junk foods or high protein foods like meat, chicken, turkey, etc. because our stomach lacks the amount of acid that requires to digest this kind of food since we were never meant to eat them in the first place. Your diet should contain 80% alkaline foods and 20% acidic foods. This means that we need moderation for some foods and for some a complete no which we don't need, find a substitute for that.

"Change Your Bad Habits By Practicing New Behaviours."

DO YOU KNOW?

The main ingredients in aerated beverages like coke, Pepsi are sugar, caffeine, phosphoric acid. All of these are highly acidic and spike blood glucose levels. If you cut your fingernails and put them into coke, the next morning they would have disappeared. Now you can imagine what they can do to your bones, teeth enamel. Switching to a whole grain diet will help you to get over this.

Health Benefits Of Alkaline Diet-

Improves Bone And Teeth Health-

As discussed earlier, when we eat acidic foods, the acidic byproduct leaches alkaline minerals like calcium from our bones. Increased acidity enhances the activity of osteoclasts(cells that degrade bones), increases the risk of osteoporosis. Now, if the diet does not lead to an acidic residue, there is no need for the bones to release calcium. So an increase in fruits and vegetables, with their alkaline residue, is great for bone structure. Studies have shown that carotenoids such as beta carotene, lycopene, lutein, and zeaxanthin can increase bone density as found in many fruits and vegetables.

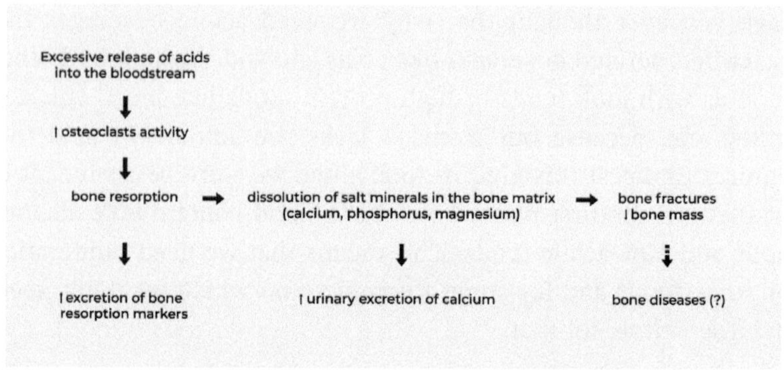

Optimizes The Immune System-

"Only the immune system can save us" we learned this in covid 19 pandemic and an alkaline diet improves your immunity. We can improve immunity by taking care of our diet. A bottle of coke has a pH value of 2.5, with around 10 tsp or more equivalent of refined sugar. To neutralize the acidic pH produced by one bottle of coke, our body requires 32 glasses of alkaline water with pH 10.No one with an alkaline body balance succumb to the covid 19 virus as in an alkaline body there is no inflammatory hyper response, and innate and adaptive immunity would be working smoothly (Dr. Eapen Koshy).

In a body with an acidic pH balance, the white blood cells which are on the frontline of our immune system and protect us from illness become lethargic and weakened. An alkaline pH of 7.4 is the perfect balance that a human body should maintain to be free of illness. A well-oxygenated alkaline balanced body has adequate immunity to successfully fight diseases. Diseases occur in a body that has low oxygenated, acidic cells as its immunity becomes weak. This happens because of a nutrient-deficient toxic diet, toxic emotions, and a toxic life. (Koshy)

Protects Against Kidney Disease-

The kidneys play an extremely important role in maintaining the body acid-base ratio by excreting nonvolatile acids and regenerating and reabsorbing bicarbonate in the kidneys' tubules. The process of trying to digest acidic food causes the breakdown of bones and muscles and leaches calcium out of the bones, which puts an excess load on the kidneys. Some of the calcium may be deposited as a stone in the kidneys, causing the further problems. People with urinary tract infections are usually given medication to make their urine alkaline to control the infection. Bacteria that cause this infection are partial to acidic medium. By making the urine alkaline, these bacteria cease to thrive. We can do this without medication by just adding an alkaline diet to our life.

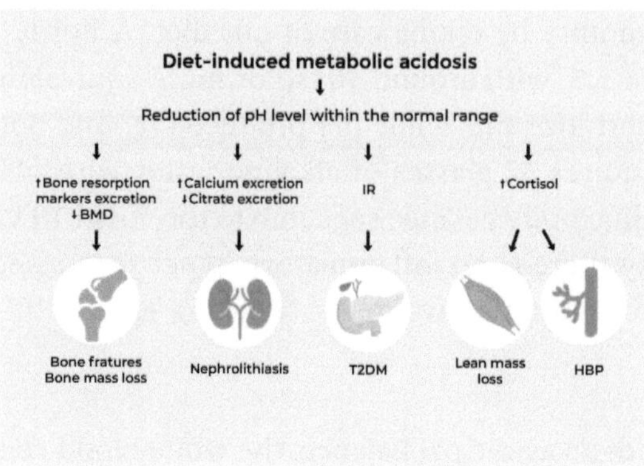

Consequences to health from low-grade metabolic acidosis induced by diet. Dietary-induced low-grade metabolic may predispose to various disorders including bone metabolism impairment, kidney stone formation, loss of lean mass, increased systemic blood pressure, and risk of type 2 diabetes mellitus.

BMD: Bone mineral density, IR: insulin resistance, T2DM: type 2 diabetes mellitus, HBP: high blood pressure. (in the figure)

Protects Against Cancer-

Cancer cells thrive and multiply in areas that are too acidic for normal cells. Keeping our body alkaline goes a long way in protecting it from cancer.

#Oil pulling- it is an ancient practice in Ayurveda, the traditional medicine system in India. Oil pulling is swishing oil around the mouth like mouthwash and then spits out.

Studies show that oil pulling reduces bacteria in the mouth. There are hundreds of different types of bacteria in the mouth. While maximum is friendly bacteria but others are not. The bacteria in your mouth creates biofilm on your teeth, a thin layer known as plaque. Having some plaque on your teeth is perfectly normal, but if it gets out of hand. It can cause various problems like cavities, gingivitis, bad breath, gum inflammation.

How does it work?

When you swish the oil around your mouth, the bacteria get swept away and dissolve in the liquid oil. People do oil pulling with any oil like sesame oil, extra virgin coconut oil. Extra virgin coconut oil is the most popular choice due to its good taste, it also has a favorable fatty acid profile, contains a high amount of lauric acid, which has antimicrobial properties.

Streptococcus mutans is one of the most common bacteria in your mouth, a key player in building plaque and tooth decay. One study in 60 adults showed that oil pulling with coconut oil for 10 minutes every day significantly reduced the number of streptococcus mutans in saliva.

HOW TO DO OIL PULLING?

1.Take one tablespoon of coconut or sesame oil in your mouth.

2.Swish the oil around your mouth for 5-10 minutes initially, gradually you can increase the timing up to 20 minutes.

3.Spit out the oil and brush your teeth.

TIP- Use neem twigs instead of a toothbrush, it has antimicrobial and antibacterial properties hence it protects your teeth against bacteria. It maintains an alkaline level in saliva, protects enamel, strengthens gums, prevents plaque, whitens teeth, and eliminates bad odor.

#How to drink tea or coffee?

Are you one of them who can't live without tea? Most people drink tea just out of habit or flavor. As I have said earlier, nothing is bad until you make it bad. Tea is not a bad thing. The problem is in the preparation method and consumption frequency. What we usually do is boil milk with tea until it darkens and waits for that strong aroma. The problem starts from here because milk modifies the biological activities of tea ingredients. Flavonoids in tea called catechins are thought to be responsible for their beneficial effects on the heart. The protein found in milk called caseins interacts with tea to reduce the concentration of catechins. And after adding milk the ingredient that makes it worse is " white sugar".Tea and coffee have antioxidant properties but they are overrated and hyped by advertisements. But do you need these, NO it's optional whether you want them or not because fruits and vegetables are not only full of antioxidants but also alkaline. Tea and coffee are grown in acidic soils, unsuitable for growing most fruits, vegetables, and grains. They Are Inherently Acidic. It raises acidic levels in the body and increases the activity of osteoclasts cells. And the food industry adds harmful chemicals in the process of tea manufacturing.

Have you ever had a headache if you don't eat vegetables or fruit one day? But this usually happens with regular tea or coffee drinkers. Why? It's called Caffeine Withdrawal Headache, it means when you drink any caffeinated drink it affects neural activity in the brain and increases alertness while reducing fatigue, caffeine narrows the blood vessels in your brain, without it your blood vessels widen. The resulting boost in blood flow could trigger a headache or result in other symptoms of withdrawal.

This happens usually to people who get dependent on caffeine and abruptly stop its consumption.

How to change this habit?

Change that comes gradually is sustainable. If you are extremely addicted like you drink 3-4 cups a day, first reduce the cups and make it 1 or 2 and switch to green tea, black tea, green coffee, black coffee. Then slowly shift to herbal teas, infusions. It's better if you try this with someone, like a challenge that makes it easier and more achievable. We'll see the recipes of substitutes for tea in the recipes section.

How has my patient cured her major acidity issue?

One day I got a call from a lady(Madhu), her brother was already in my weight loss batch. She started talking about how badly she wanted to lose weight because she wanted to become a makeup artist and she wanted to look slim trim, during the conversation she told me about her acid reflux, constipation, bloating, headache, low blood pressure, lethargy, swelling(whole body including face).

She uses to take medicines for headaches (crocin), acidity for the last 15 years, and only one thing changed in those 15 years that her problem increased. She use to walk for 30-35 minutes occasionally. When she came to me, I told her to do one thing from day one and that was eliminating the milk tea (strong), and if she wants something hot to drink then take green tea or infusion tea(best).In the first 7 days, she had headaches, acid reflux(some concoctions and infused teas helped her to overcome the issues), one more thing I wanna add is she didn't take any medicine during this period, after one week the acid reflux issue got a bit better so as headache, she continued her normal diet for 1 month, after 1 month the body started showing positive results her energy level increased, acidity, bloating, swelling significantly decreased and most importantly she was able to move more in comparison to earlier and the "feel-good" factor came. Now, you must be thinking, is this a joke that she was taking pills for 15 years but nothing improved, in fact, the symptoms got worse and she eliminated tea and got better.

Yes, that's true she only eliminated "one" thing that was increasing acidic levels in the body, the main culprit behind the series of symptoms. See, your body has everything to heal itself, the only thing it needs is you stop putting things inside that worsen the condition. So, coming back to her journey, she lost 10 kg in 3 months, the best part was that she got medicine free. She came for weight loss but when she left the batch after achieving the goal she was happier for the fact that she doesn't need to pop a pill for acidity, headache, or any churan for clear bowel movement. We don't realize that it's not normal to pop a pill every day without knowing how long this will continue.

 # Fasting(yes, it's back in town)

What is fasting?

Fasting(Upvas)in Sanskrit has two words which mean "upa" means near-"vas" means sitting.Up+vas means to stay next to ourselves or the divine spark within, self-realization.

People do fasting for various reasons like for religious or spiritual reasons, to lose weight, to detox body, some common names of fasting are Ramadan, Ekadashi, partial fasting, absolute fasting, intermittent fasting, dry fasting, lent, Navratri. The way of doing fast also has so many variations like there are fasts in which food is completely restricted, in some you can drink only water, while in modern-day fasting involves NO to specific foods like no-carb fast and so on.

Earlier people use to do fast based on moon cycles and other religious reasons in different cultures that we know also and it is called traditional fasting. Nowadays, modern fasting has also come into our lives for weight loss, or to achieve any short-term body goals. Fasting has an immense role in immunity, according to research fasting kick starts stem cells into producing new white blood cells, which fight off infection. Fasting "flips a regenerative switch" which prompts stem cells to create brand new WBC's, essentially regenerating the entire immune system.

Prolonged fasting reduces the enzyme PKA, which is linked to aging and a hormone that increases cancer risk and tumor growth. When you starve, the immune system tries to save energy and one of the things it can do to save energy is to recycle a lot of the immune cells that are not needed, especially those that may be damaged. Scientists say that prolonged fasting appears to shift stem cells of the immune system from a dormant state to an active state of self-renewal. Once you start eating again, your stem cells kick back into high gear to replenish the cells that were recycled.

Another good thing about fasting is that the body rids itself "of the parts of the system that might be damaged or old, the inefficient parts, during the fasting.

Have you ever heard about water fasting for 3 days?

This is the practice whereby you do not eat or drink anything for three days, water fast usually lasts for 24 hours to 72 hours(you can drink water).

There is another popular fasting called “intermittent fasting”.Intermittent fasting is the eating practice that revolves around periods of eating and fasting. Under intermittent fasting, people go through an extended fasting period and they have a few short hours of eating(feeding window)where they can eat.

The most popular form of intermittent fasting:-

1.Fasting window-16 hours, feeding window-8 hours
2.Fasting window-12 hours, feeding window -12 hours
3.Fasting window-18 hours, feeding window-6 hours
4.Fasting window-14 hours, feeding window-10 hours

If you want to do fasting for the first time, start with intermittent fasting and then can go for water fasting for 3 days if all goes smoothly and it’s always better to do this under guidance.

 # Add variations in a workout regime

I do this religiously, I get bored if I do the same exercise daily it’s like you are eating the same food daily. Exercise variations not only add interest but also improve performance and decrease injury. It is important to apply variations correctly to maximize results. If you are an exercise enthusiast and looking for performance improvement the phenomenon called “Adaptive resistance” can stand in the way of improved performance. Adaptive resistance is when you have done an exercise over a long period of time, and your body no longer responds to it. It can cause injury too. This happens because if you do the same exercise for a prolonged period, you use the same muscles in the same pattern/angle which causes more wear and tear on the same soft tissue structure.

Creating variations and changing exercises in your routine can create a new stimulus, which creates more progress over time. And if you rotate or exercise every so often, your injury risk will decrease. Now moderation is the word to remember when creating variations in regime because too many variations can also become an issue. When choosing exercises for your regime, two to three variations should be chosen for each muscle or movement. If more exercises are performed, it becomes more difficult to adapt because you are always doing something different and waking up the system.

Are you one of those who think that exercise only melts your fat or makes you slim? Then you are wrong because it does way more than this, it can improve your memory, concentration, and much more.

We know that when we exercise our blood flow increases, and we feel more positive and happy because when we exercise the body releases endorphins(the feel-good hormone).

Some studies show that exercise subconsciously affects our brain much more than this. Your brain is like plastic, in the sense that every stimulus/input can mold and reshape your brain throughout your lifetime. At a neurobiological level, this reshaping comes from neurogenesis(the creation of new neurons/nerve cells) and neuroplasticity(the growth and improvements of neural networks)

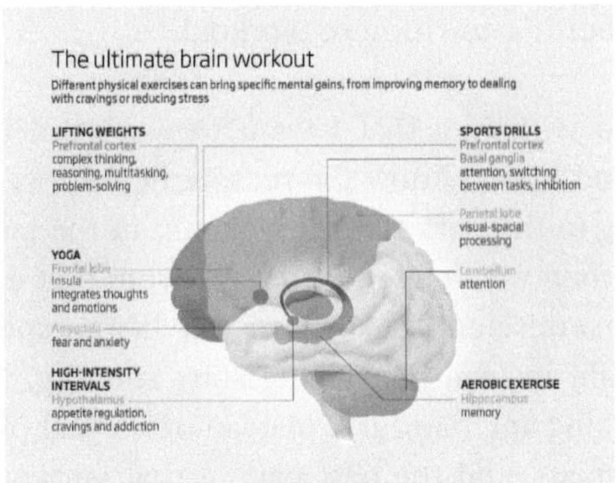

My personal experience about variations in exercise-

In 2020, I came back to my home from Delhi due to the covid-19 pandemic like many others. When I came back I started an exercise regime which I followed for months, the pattern of my exercise was like 30 minutes walk,10 minutes animal walk,2 minutes plank, then I use to do pull-ups for 5-10 minutes, removing congress grass from the park was also the part of my workout routine(my mother maintains this park which has an area about 2.5 acres, she use to remove the unwanted and allergic grass by hands, gardening tools).

But after some time (2-3 months) I started losing interest in workouts, I started making excuses with myself for not going like it's too hot today, I have other important work, etc. But I had that guilt that I'm not working out daily and properly and this I could feel because I have felt that feeling of satisfaction and feel-good factor that comes out after working out(that moment when sweat makes you happy and satiated). But it's true if you want something, nothing can stop you(sounds dramatic but it's so true; law of attraction), my brother who lives in Bangalore came for holidays at home, he is a fitness freak he loves everything about being fit whether it's nutrition or workout.

So, I discussed with him that I want to work out but I'm losing interest in it and I don't know the reason, he said we'll go together in the morning to the park when I woke up in the morning he was ready already then we went and trust me from that day I got a new definition of exercise and the reason was his perspective towards exercise, he said instead of walking start running, that day I did squats(so amazing and painful), instead of normal plank I did side plank, sumo squats, and the best part of that workout regime was a race with brother(its so good to explore this kind of workout; an exercise in a community or with your family member). When we came home I was refreshed and energetic, I learned one thing from him that you should be experimenting in exercise if you will stick to one pattern it's not sustainable. And I'm following this till now, adding variations in a workout has become part of it.

#Don't put supplements inside the body blindly

"I can't have this, but I can take supplements of it" I often face this. It's always best if you can get your macronutrients and micronutrients through your diet, if you are not able to get it from due to any reason(should be valid and sensible), only then you should get it from a supplement.

Let's take a simple example if your test showed that your vitamin-D is very low, you should take a vitamin d supplement but under the guidance of your doctor so that you will get to know when to stop it otherwise it can cause toxicity, with supplementation take sunbath regularly as I have already mentioned. Do you know? According to data, Indians bought over 500 crore pills of vitamin c, zinc, multivitamins to battle covid in 2020, sales of zinc supplement Zincovit increased by 93% with a total of 54 crore tablets sold in 2020 while that of vitamin -C grew 110% with around 185 crore pills being sold, a growth of over 100% when compared to 2019.

Why did sales zoom?

People rushed to buy these pills to protect against the fast-spreading covid-19. While zinc deficiency has been linked to higher severity of covid infection, consumption of vitamin C has been associated with higher immunity and reduction in oxidative stress that can be caused by covid.

Vitamin-D sales also increased, the role of vitamin d3, also known as calcifediol, has been linked to reduced risk of severe infection, and even death, in covid-19 patients.

Can we get these nutrients only from supplements?

NO, you can get these nutrients in sufficient amounts from your diet only, you need supplements when you are severely deficient, during pregnancy, etc. Otherwise, normally your food is capable of giving you an adequate amount of these nutrients.

You don't need those expensive and high dosages of vitamin c or other nutrients. Why? I'll tell you.

Have you ever read the composition of the tablet of vitamin C, No? It contains only ascorbic acid(it's just a part of vitamin c, you need vitamin-C complex). Vitamin -C complex will help you in optimizing your immunity not only ascorbic acid(that too in high dosage). If you have problems like varicose veins and hemorrhoids, your problem will increase because of ascorbic acid consumption in high dosage.

Vitamin-C complex contains-

1.Rutin(vitamin P) is one of the flavonoids, also called bioflavonoids, and strengthens blood vessels and other collagen-containing tissues.

2. "K" factor supports the clotting mechanism of the blood.

3. "J" factor supports the oxygen-carrying capacity of the blood, which is important for all the cells.

4.Tyrosinase(as organic copper)is a trace element activator.

5. Ascorbic acid as an antioxidant is (a)part of the naturally

occurring vitamin-C complex. It functions to preserve the fragile rutin, other bioflavonoids, and the complex.

Some great food sources of vitamin-C-

Red pepper(½ cup)- 95mg
Broccoli,cooked(1 cup)-74mg
Kiwi(1 medium)- 70mg
Indian gooseberry/Amla(100g)-700mg
Seabuckthorn(100g)-695mg

I guess you got the idea of consuming the nutrients from food is always better than having supplements and if you are consuming any supplement read the label and be mindful about what you are taking. So that you can't say that "I'm taking a supplement then why I'm deficient" and another factor is how much your body is absorbing it (bioavailability).

Info fact-

Animals can make vitamin C by themselves, humans can't that's why we need it daily in our diet. Do you think that a high dosage will give you more vitamin C, NO the body will absorb the required amount and the rest will pass out through your urine, so you are buying expensive urine. The best way to get it is to eat it vitamin C in small portion throughout the day.

 # Utensils role in your health-

Did you know that cooking in some utensils can be dangerous for your health?

I know we all want a modular kitchen with decent cookware that looks beautiful to your eyes. Utensils play a major role when it comes to healthy food. I want you to know how your utensils create health issues like hormonal imbalance(a major issue in females these days), cancer, thyroid, etc.

Heres list of toxic cookwares -

1.ALUMINIUM- you may find this ideal cookware because it's lightweight, strong, versatile, recyclable but the reality is a bit bitter. Aluminum is a neurotoxic metal which means it's harmful to your nervous system. Studies have shown that elevated levels of aluminum metal in the body cause central nervous system diseases like Alzheimer's, amyotrophic lateral sclerosis, Parkinson's dementia.

Aluminum heats very quickly and reacts with acidic vegetables and foods like tomato, vinegar, and citrus. Cooking in aluminum utensils is not advisable.

"The higher the temperature, the more the leaching. The foil that we use is not suitable for cooking and is not suitable for packing food".Without heating, there will be no leaching of aluminum in food.

Aluminum Accumulation Effect On Bones-

High aluminum levels in the body alter bone mineralization, matrix formation, as well as parathyroid and bone cell activity. Ironically, one of the most common signs of excessive aluminum accumulation is hypercalcemia or high calcium levels in the blood.

This happens because the presence of aluminum impedes calcium deposition in bones, thus leading to elevated blood calcium levels. As a result, PTH secretion, the hormone secreted by the parathyroid gland. Additionally, chronic aluminum toxicity greatly reduces the osteoblast(responsible for new bone formation) population and inhibits bone mineralization, resulting in osteoporosis.

2.Teflon(non-stick cookware)- People choose nonstick material because it's convenient and ubiquitous but it also tops the list when it comes to most dangerous utensils.

The chemical behind this nonstick property of Teflon is the coating of PTFE(polytetrafluoroethylene), which is a plastic polymer that starts to leach toxins when heated above 572 degrees Fahrenheit.

Another chemical compound found in Teflon cookware is PFOA(perfluorooctanoic acid), which has been linked to several cancers including breast, prostate, ovarian cancer.

3.Plastic- if you use plastic utensils that come with your microwave, it's time to change because it is the worst. The evidence is mounting that plastic food containers are bad for our health. The two key culprits are the man-made chemicals Phthalates and Bisphenol A(BPA) which are often added to plastic to help it keep its shape and pliability, known as "endocrine disruptors" these substances have been found to affect hormones, such as estrogen and testosterone which can cause reproductive and other health issues.

The healthiest options to cook in -

1.Cast-iron
2. Stainless steel(high quality)
3.Clay
4.Ceramic
5.Glass based utensils

#Spend some time with nature

Yes, connect with nature, mud to grow your microbiome of the gut. Don't stop your kids from playing with mud, because this will make their immune system strong. Yes, you read that right. Excess cleanliness is decreasing our immunity. Asthma and allergies are higher in wealthy countries due to a lack of exposure to bacteria and other microorganisms. Have you ever noticed the kids who live in slums? They don't live in clean and sanitized, due to which they get exposed to the bacterias, communicable diseases at an early age and develops stronger immunity, that helps them to ward off the diseases later in life, this phenomenon is called "immune training".

In a study, based on analysis of data until 29th July 2020, more than 5 lakh deaths had been reported- more than 70% of it in high-income countries. People in rich countries have better access to healthcare and vaccines, and things like clean drinking water, due to which they remain safer from infectious disease, which leads to a weaker immune system. Cleanliness is good but it should not be done in excess like choose less harsh floor cleaners and don't use one for a long time keep changing it alternatively, do not use sanitizer if you are at a place where you can use handwash. Stay connected with the dirt of your garden.

Soil and the human gut contain approximately the same number of active microorganisms, while human gut microbiome diversity is only 10% of the soil biodiversity and has decreased dramatically with the modern lifestyle.

We don't have a garden, how we will do this?

Yes, I can relate to this in cities we have high-rise buildings with no such facilities, you can buy organic soil put that in a pot, and play with it with your kids for 20-25 minutes, make structures, or anything that you like. "Don't think about your nails, you can clean them later with lemon". Play some relaxing music, enjoy that moment.

Gardening is another best option, our body loves the tuning with nature.

#Listen to your doctors but don't follow them blindly.

"My doctor says you can eat everything, just take these medicines regularly".If you follow this pattern, you're making the biggest mistake of your life and creating your problems. How is this possible, that you can eat anything? It's not the way to cure a disease, food(nutrition) is the fuel that you are taking by birth, medicines cant replace the value of it. Take medicine if you need it, but keep a check on your diet if you don't want to get dependent on that medicine. For example, if you have hypothyroidism and you are taking medicine for the last 10-15 years, don't you think something is wrong with the process. And don't say that it's irreversible because it is reversible.

#Don't make excuses

I never saw this much shortage of coconut water ever in life that I saw in the covid-19 period. Instead of cold drinks people were drinking coconut water, orange juice. It's nothing like that we can't do it, the thing is that we don't understand the value of it. We wait for the extreme, and then we take action against it. This journey of a healthy lifestyle will not only give you a healthy body but also the new you, the best of you. Because food is related to your mind, body, and soul. Don't listen to what others are saying, listen to your body.

In starting you may dislike the change but don't stop because good things take time to come, stay dedicated to what you have started.

CHAPTER VI

Recipe

Substitutes are a must in a healthy lifestyle. Sharing some amazing, delicious yet healthy recipes.

Infusions/ Herbal Tea-

1.Peppermint tea

Method-

Put 15-20 peppermint leaves in 1 glass of boiling water and allow it to seep for 10-15 min, serve it lukewarm.

2.Curry leaves tea-

Method-

Boil 10-15 curry leaves in 1 glass of water for 5-7 minutes, strain, and serve it lukewarm.

3.Infusion(best for acidity,bloating,acid reflux)-

Put 1 teaspoon fennel seeds, cumin seeds(1 tsp), bishop's weed(½ tsp) into a pan, pour 1.5 glasses of water into it and boil till it reduces to half, strain it and serve it lukewarm.

4.Liquorice and thyme infusion

Method-

Brew both ingredients in 1 glass of water for 5-7 minutes, serve it lukewarm.

The method of infusions or herbal tea will be the same. Don't drink any infusion too hot or too cold, drink it lukewarm or warm. Here is the list of other combinations to make infusions using the same method-

- Tulsi+ fennel seeds+green cardamom.
- Tulsi+srilankan rolled cinnamon + raw grated turmeric.
- Ginger+ tulsi+turmeric
- Bay leaf+ Srilankan rolled cinnamon
- Black cardamom+ cloves
- Lemongrass+ turmeric+ green cardamom
- Nutmeg powder+saffron strands+khus khus
- Nutmeg powder+fennel seeds+ cinnamon stick
- Mint+ fennel seeds+ peppercorns
- Blue tea(butterfly pea flower tea)
- Chamomile tea
- Kahwa

Try these variations and the recipes that your grandmother, mother use to make.

Other options(secondary)- Matcha tea, Black tea(add fennel seeds,green cardamom,tulsi).

SMOOTHIES-

Smoothies are the best options when it comes to consuming fruits and vegetables with a twist. You can mix and match according to season, region, availability.

Green smoothie

Ingredients-

1.Spinach/kale/celery/lettuce/curry leaves/(1big handful)
2.Green or red apple diced(1 cup)
3.Wheatgrass
4.Lemon juice(1 tablespoon)
5.Coconut water
6.Roasted flaxseed powder(½ teaspoon)

Method-

Blend everything together except flaxseed powder, sprinkle flaxseed powder while serving.

Dark choco smoothie

Ingredients

1.Cacao powder(2 tablespoons)
2.Coconut milk/cashew milk/almond milk/soy milk(1.5 cups)
3.Dates(4 pitted)
4.Green cardamom(¼ teaspoon)optional

Method-

Blend everything together, and serve

Banana fig delight

Ingredient

1.Banana(1)
2.Fresh figs diced(2)

3.Dates(4 pitted)
4.Any plant-based milk(1.5 cups)
5.Soaked chia seeds(1 teaspoon)

Method-

Blend everything together, except chia seeds, add chia seeds while serving.

Plain carrot smoothie

Ingredient
1.Carrots(2)
2.Black pepper(2 freshly cracked)
3. Virgin coconut oil(1 tablespoon)
4.Lemon(1 teaspoon)

Method-

Blend everything together, serve it.

(good option in the journey of immune system optimization, must add in diet)

Sapodilla(chikoo)smoothie

Ingredient
1.Sapodilla(5)
2.Coconut milk(1.5 cup)
3.Green cardamom powder(1 teaspoon)

Method

Blend everything together, and serve it.

Beetroot smoothie

Ingredients

1.Beetroot diced(½)
2.Apple diced(1)
3.Ginger(1 coin)
4.Pomegranate(3 tablespoons)
5.Lemon(1 tablespoon)

Method

Blend everything together, and serve it.

INFUSED WATER-

Good quality hydration is important.

Orange peel infused water

Ingredients

1. Orange or any citrus fruit (1)
2. 1-liter water
3. Mint leaves(10-20)

Method

Peel off the skin of the orange, add the peel, mint in water, sip on it.

Star anise fennel seeds infused water

Ingredient

1.Star anise (1)

2. 1-liter water

3.Fennel seeds(1 tablespoon)

Method

Add the ingredients to water, keep it for 15 minutes and then sip on it.

Cinnamon-black cardamom infused water

Ingredient

1.Srilankan rolled cinnamon stick(½ inch)

2.Black cardamom(1)

3. 1-liter water

Method

Put the ingredients in water, keep it for 15-20 minutes, sip on it.

Basil seeds infused water

Ingredients

1.Basil seeds(1 teaspoon)

2.Lemon slices

3. 1-liter water

Method

Add the ingredients to water, let the basil seeds swell, sip on it.

Tulsi/curry leaves infused water

Ingredients

1. Tulsi leaves/curry leaves(20 leaves)
2. Cucumber slices
3. 1-liter water

Method

Put all the ingredients in water, keep aside for 1 hour, sip on it.

Carrot-mint infused water

Ingredients

1. Sliced carrots(2)
2. Fennel seeds(1 tablespoon)
3. Mint leaves(15-20)

Method

Add the ingredients in water, leave aside for 1 hour, and it's ready.

Note- Do not consume infused water after lunchtime because when you drink infused water you may urinate more so it's best to finish it before lunchtime. And consume it within 2-3 hours.

BREAKFAST OPTIONS

Quinoa poha

Ingredients

1. Quinoa(1 cup)
2. Tomato(1)
3. Onion(1)
4. Carrot(1)
5. Capsicum(1)
6. Potatoes(½)
7. Mustard oil
8. Mustard seeds
9. Curry leaves
10. Spice mix(½ tsp)
11. Rocksalt

Method

To cook quinoa- in a pan, add mustard oil and roast quinoa until it starts popping, add 1.5 cup water and let it boil for 15 minutes.

To make poha- in a pan, add mustard oil, mustard seeds, curry leaves, and all the vegetables, saute them for 2 min, add the spice mix, salt, after 5-7 minutes add boiled quinoa, mix well and switch off the flame after 2 min, you can add lemon while serving it.

Red rice poha sprout mix(Serves 2)

Ingredient

1.Red rice poha(1 cup)
2.Diced vegetables(1.5 cup)

3. Mustard seeds(1 teaspoon)
4.Green chilies to taste
5.Turmeric(¼ teaspoon)
6.Rocksalt or sea salt to taste
7.Roasted peanuts(10-20)
8.Cashew nuts and raisins(10-15)
9.Curry leaves(10-20)
10.Coriander leaves
11.Lemon juice(2 tablespoons)
12.Grated coconut(2 tablespoon)

Method

Wash the poha in a strainer and keep it aside. Meanwhile, put a pan on flame, add mustard oil, and mustard seeds once they start popping, add curry leaves and all the diced vegetables. Add salt, turmeric. After 5 minutes, add soaked pour, cashews, raisins, and mix well 2-3 minutes. Switch off the flame and add roasted peanuts. Add lemon and garnish with grated coconut and coriander.

To make it more nutrient-dense add boiled or steamed sprouts.

Oats idli and coconut chutney

Ingredient
1.Roasted rolled oats(1 cup)
2.Rava or semolina(¾ cup)
3.Curd or yogurt(1 cup)
4.Fruit salt(1 teaspoon)
5.Water (as required)
6.Grated carrots (2)
7.Coriander leaves chopped
8.Green chili
9.Salt

10.Grated zucchini(1)

Method

Blend the oats to a fine flour. In a large bowl add semolina, powdered oats, and other ingredients mix them well, and keep them aside for 20 minutes. After 20 minutes batter looks thick add some water and fruit salt, mix it gently, grease idli molds and pour the batter into it and place it in the steamer.

Coconut chutney

Ingredients

1.Chopped fresh coconut(1 cup)
2.Green chilies (4-5)
3.Salt(as per taste)
4.Ginger (1 coin)
5.Water

Method

Blend all the above ingredients in a blender to make a fine paste.

For tempering-1 tablespoon coconut oil, mustard seeds, ¼ tsp chana dal,¼ white urad dal, curry leaves.

Method(tadka)

Heat 1 tablespoon oil in a small pan, add mustard seeds, chana dal, urad dal, and curry leaves. Add this tadka to the chutney.

Authentic south Indian idli/dosa

Ingredient

1.Unpolished red rice(4 cups)
2.Whole black gram/Urad dal(1 cup)

3.Fenugreek seeds(1 teaspoon)
4.Salt to taste

Method

Separately soak the red rice and the dal for 8-12 hours. Soak 1 teaspoon of fenugreek seeds with dal. Add salt to taste.Grind the soaked rice in the blender till you get a slightly coarse(but almost smooth)paste. Pour into a large bowl. Grind the soaked urad dal in the blender till very smooth and mix with the rice paste.

Allow the mixture to ferment for 8-12 hours depending on the room temperature. In summer,6-7 hours is sufficient, but on cooler days it takes longer. Pour into an idli steamer to make idlis. Add water to achieve the consistency of dosa batter to make dosas.Make dosas on cast iron tawa instead of non-stick, grease the Tawa with half chopped potato or onion, do not pour the oil on Tawa just put some oil on the potato and grease the Tawa with it.

Variations

You can make uttapam/chilla from the same batter by adding chopped or grated vegetables. Serve it with coconut or peanut chutney and sambhar.

Pessaruttu

Ingredient
1.Whole moong dal(1 cup)
2.Rice(½ cup)
3.Salt to taste
4.Water
5.Green chili
6.Ginger(1 coin)

7.Coriander leaves

Method

Soak moong dal and rice separately overnight. Next morning put all the above ingredients in a blender to make a fine paste. Grease the cast-iron Tawa and make dosas. Serve it with coconut chutney.

Variations

You can add vegetables to the batter like grated carrots, tomato, grated cabbage, onion, grated pumpkin to make it more nutrient-dense.

Sprouts chaat

Ingredients

1.Any type of boiled and steamed sprouts(1 cup)
2.Grated or steamed carrots(1)
3.Diced capsicum(1)
4.Tomatoes(1)
5.Green chili
6.Diced cucumber(1)
7.Grated zucchini(1)
8.Salt
9.Lemon(2 tablespoon)
10.Coriander leaves
12.Steamed broccoli(3-4 florets)optional

Method

Add boiled or steamed sprouts in a large bowl, all the above ingredients, and toss it. Serve it fresh.

Variations

You can add boiled and cooled diced potato to sprouts.

(Boiled and cooled potatoes are a good source of resistant starch).

Ragi porridge

Ingredient

1.Ragi flour(4 tablespoon)
2.Date paste(2 tablespoon)
3.Fresh grated coconut(¼ cup)/coconut milk(½ cup)/dessicated coconut(2 tablespoons)

Method

Mix the ragi with 1 cup cold water till there are no lumps and cook for about 5 minutes on a medium flame till the ragi is cooked. Stir briskly throughout because ragi flour tends to form lumps. You will know it's done when its color changes to a deep brown. Add the date paste and turn off the flame. Top with coconut milk or coconut and serve.

Variations-

Ragi can be replaced with cracked wheat or whole or rolled oats. Cinnamon and cardamom can be used to enhance flavor.

Refreshing Drinks

Sattu and mint drink(ideal option for refreshment)

Ingredients

1.Sattu(3 tablespoons)
2.Cumin seeds powder(½ tsp)
3.Black salt

4.Mint leaves(5-6)
5.Lemon(1.5 tablespoon)
6.Coriander leaves (few)
7. 1 glass of water

Method

Blend all the above ingredients in a blender jar and serve it.

Lemon mint drink

Ingredient
1.Lemon(2 tablespoons)
2.Mint leaves(5-8)
3.Black salt
4.Soaked chia seeds(1 teaspoon)
5.Peppercorn(1 freshly cracked)
6. 1 glass of water

Method

In a blender, add mint, lemon, black salt, freshly cracked peppercorn, water, and blend it. Add soaked chia seeds while serving.

SALADS-

Super salad

Ingredients
1. Diced tomato(1 medium)

2.Steamed mushroom(5)
3. 1 carrot(steamed or grated)
4.Steamed peas(5 tablespoons)
5.Sprouted and boiled moong dal(2 tablespoons)
6.Chopped onion(1)
7.Black roasted sesame seeds(½ tsp)
8.Peppercorns(2-3 freshly cracked)
9.Sea salt
10. Grated Indian gooseberry/amla(1 tsp)

Method

In a large bowl put all the vegetables, sprouts, add pepper, salt, and grated amla, toss it well. Serve it fresh.

Millet and mixed vegetable salad(serves 6)

Ingredients
1. Foxtail millet(2 cups)
2.Boiled water(2.5 cups)
3.Black raisins(¼ cup)
4.Green and red bell peppers(½ cup)
5.Minced onion(¼ cup)
6.Boiled green peas(¼ cup)
7.Celery finely chopped(¼ cup)
8.Mint, finely chopped(¼ cup)
9.Lemon juice(1 tablespoon)
10.Black pepper(½ teaspoon freshly cracked)
11.Salt to taste
12. Romaine lettuce for garnishing on serving plate (50g)

Method

Soak the millet for 2-8 hours.Drain.Cook in 4 cups of water in a pot or pressure cooker. It should not be mushy. Mix all other ingredients and fluff with a fork. Add the cooked millet. Garnish with romaine lettuce.

Variation

Any millet can be used in place of foxtails like a barnyard, Kodo,proso, or little millet.

Zoodles

Ingredients

1.Carrots(1)
2.Zucchini(2)
3.Mint leaves
4.Salt
5.Pepper
6.Spiralizer
7.Black roasted sesame seeds

Method

Make zoodles of zucchini and carrots using a spiralizer. Add all the ingredients to it and garnish it with mint.

Variation

You can use homemade tomato chutney to get a tangy taste.

Tip- You can lightly steam or saute your salad vegetables if you have any digestion problems like heaviness after eating raw salad. If you are eating salad with a meal, do not add dressing, salt, or pepper, but you can go for dressing if you're taking salad as a meal replacement. You can add different vegetables, nuts, seeds to your salad like raw grated papaya, black or golden raisins, alfalfa sprouts, fenugreek sprouts, mint, tulsi, cashew nuts.

Dressings

Tahini

Ingredients

1.Sesame seeds(3 tablespoons)

2.Salt to taste

3.Water(2 teaspoons)

4.Olive oil(1 teaspoon)

Method

Roast the sesame seeds on medium to low heat until slightly brown. Once cool, transfer it to the grinder, add salt, grind it for a few seconds, add water and oil, and grind again, tahini is ready.

Green hummus

Ingredients

1.Sprouted and boiled green chickpeas(30 g)

2.Salt to taste

3.Garlic cloves(2)

4.Tahini mix(3 tablespoons)

5.Olive oil(1 tablespoon)

6.Green chili (1)

7.Lemon juice(1 tablespoon)

Method

Put all the ingredients in the grinder except oil, once ground add oil and blend once again, it's ready.

Mayonnaise

Ingredients

1.Soaked cashews(½ cup)

2.Chopped onions(2 tablespoons)

3.Lime juice(1 tablespoon)
4.Garlic clove(1 small)
5.Salt to taste
6.Pepper to taste
7.Mustard to taste

Method

Blend the ingredients together. Add1/4 cup of water a little at a time to make a smooth paste.

You can flavor the mayonnaise with any herbs, celery, or red pepper while blending.

LUNCH OPTIONS

Moringa khichdi

Ingredients

1.Cauliflower
2.Beans
3.Peas
4.Carrot
5.Sonamasuri rice(500g)
6.Moong dal(50g)
7.Turmeric powder(½ tsp)
8.Black pepper powder(½ tsp)
9.Green chili(1)
10.Salt to taste
11.Moringa powder(2 tsp)
12.Mustard oil(1 tablespoon)
13.Cumin seeds(1 tsp)

Method

In a pressure cooker put mustard oil, add cumin seeds, and all the chop[ped vegetables, dal, rice, moringa powder. Saute it for 2-3 minutes and water accordingly. Close the lid and let it pressure cook for three to four whistles. Top it with 1 tablespoon cow ghee and enjoy it with curd and salad.

Variations

You can add green leafy vegetables, soaked garden cress seeds in curd, moringa leaves, drumsticks, lentils, fenugreek seeds as tadka, capsicum, tomato.

Nutritious chapatis

Ingredients

1.Whole wheat flour(1 cup)

2.Oats flour(½ cup)

3.Besan(½ cup)

4.Maze flour/Makki flour(½ cup)

5.Ragi flour(½ cup)

6.Beetroot/bottle gourd/pumpkin/spinach/moringa leaves/ carrots.

7.Water

8.Ghee

Method

In a large bowl, add the vegetable of your choice. If you are adding spinach, blend it in a blender and then mix it with flour. Add these vegetables in any form. The ratio should be 1:1 of vegetables and flour.

This method will increase the taste and nutrition value of chapatis. Eat these healthy chapatis with any sabzi or dal.

Dry vegetable dish

Ingredients

1. 1/2kg Mixed vegetables finely chopped into cubes(you can use capsicum, carrots, french beans, potatoes, onions, cauliflower)

2.Grated coconut(2 -4 tablespoons)

For tempering

1.Mustard seeds(1 tsp)

2.Asafoetida(a pinch)

3.Ginger-chilli paste to taste

4.Curry leaves(2-3)

5.Sal to taste

6.Turmeric powder(½ tsp)

Method

Steam the mixed vegetables. In a heated pan, add the mustard seeds. When the mustard seeds splutter, turn off the flame, add the asafoetida, and then turmeric and dry roast. When the smell permeates, add the curry leaves and finally mix in the steamed vegetables, ginger-chili paste, salt, and fresh coconut. Mix well and serve hot.

Variations

You can add crushed peanuts or roasted crushed sesame seeds instead of the grated coconut or in addition to it.

Daliya khichdi

Ingredients

1.Roasted wheat daliya(1 cup)

2.Arhar dal(3 tablespoons)

3.Split moong dal(3 tablespoons)

4.Masoor dal(3 tablespoons)

5.Sama rice(1 tablespoon)

6.Mustard oil(1 tablespoon)
7.Desi ghee(1 tablespoon)
8.Cumin seeds(1 teaspoon)
9.Water
10.Salt, spice mix, green chili, turmeric powder to taste.

Method

In a pressure cooker heat oil, add cumin seeds and other ingredients. Saute it for 1 minute and add water depending on the consistency you like. Cook for 3 whistles.

Top it with ghee and serve with curd and salad.

DINNER OPTIONS

Green papaya soup

Ingredients

1.Green papaya(1)
2. Coconut milk(2 cups)
3.Water (3 cups)
4.Lemongrass stalks(3)
5.Coriander seeds(2 tablespoons)
6.Green chili(½)
7.Black pepper powder(¼ tsp)
8.Ginger(1 coin)
9.Lemon juice(1 tablespoon)
10.Salt to taste

Method

Peel, cut, and steam the papaya until it is soft. Meanwhile, take a shallow pan, and dry roast the green chili, coriander seeds, ginger, and lemongrass together. Add some water, and let it cook till the flavors are soaked in. Add this mixture to a blender along with your steamed papaya, water, coconut milk, pepper, lemon juice, and salt. Blend and serve. Garnish with coriander leaves/seeds/nuts or whatever you like.

Broccoli soup

Ingredients

1.Chopped broccoli(2 cups)
2.Chopped potatoes(1 cup)
3.Water(3 cups)
4.Ginger(1 coin)
5.Black pepper(¼ tsp)
6.Coconut milk(1 cup)
7.Salt
8.Steamed carrot(1 large)
9.Coriander leaves
10.Pumpkin seeds(1 tablespoon)

Method

In a pan boil, the broccoli, carrots, and potatoes for 10-15 minutes, add the ginger to the pan and cook for another 2 minutes. Let the vegetables cool down and then add them to a blender and blend till it gains a smooth texture.

Pour the soup into a heated pan, add salt, pepper, coconut milk, and mix well. Pour this hot soup into a serving bowl and garnish it with coriander leaves and pumpkin seeds.

Barley and sprouts khichdi

Ingredients

1. Barley broken daliya (1 cup)
2. Moong sprout(1 cup)
3. Chopped onion(1 cup)
4. Chopped tomatoes(1 cup)
5. Mustard oil(1 tablespoon)
6. Salt to taste
7. Ghee(1 tablespoon)
8. Cumin seeds(1 tsp)
9. Water(4 glasses)
10. Green chili (2)

Method

In a pressure cooker, heat 1 tbsp oil, add cumin seeds and onion, once it starts turning light brown, add daliya, and roast it. Once the daliya is roasted add sprouts and tomatoes. Add water, salt, spice mix, and turmeric powder. Now bring the mixture to a boil, once it starts to boil, cover the lid and cook for 3-4 whistles. Serve hot and top it with ghee.

HOMEMADE PROBIOTICS

Rice kanji

Ingredients

1. Mud pot
2. Cooked rice
3. Water

4.Salt as required (optional)

Method

1.Soak ½ cup cooked rice in ½ cup water in a mud pot for about 10-12 hours or overnight.

2.Next morning, add salt (optional) to it.

3.Have this rice and water(rice kanji) in the morning on an empty stomach.

Carrot kanji

Ingredient

1.Carrots (4 orange/red)

2.Beetroot (1)

3.Mustard seeds (3-4 tbsp)

4.Salt(1 tbsp)

5.Chilli powder

6.Turmeric(¼ tsp)

7.Black pepper(4 crushed)

8.Water(3-4 liters)

Method

1.In a clay pot take carrots and beetroot.

2.Add 3-4 tbsp coarse mustard seeds.

3.Add salt to taste.

4.Add chili powder, turmeric powder, black pepper(crushed)

5.Add 3-4 liters of water.

6.Keep this in the sunlight for 4-5 days, it’s ready.

Mix vegetable pickle

Ingredients

1.Take vegetables like cucumber, beans, carrots, radish, cabbage, cauliflower, peas, beetroot, chili, garlic, onion.

2.Salt

3.White vinegar(1 cup)

4.Apple cider vinegar(1 cup)

5.Rice vinegar(½ cup)

6.Coconut sugar(3 tbsp)

7.Mustard seeds(2 tbsp)

8.Fennel seeds(1 tbsp)

9.Black pepper powder(½ tsp)

10.Caram seeds(½ tsp)

11.Turmeric powder(½ tsp)

12.Sesame seeds(1 tbsp)

Method

1.Add vegetables to a bowl, add salt and toss the vegetables.

2.Keep aside for 30 minutes to 3 hours.

3.Wash off the excess salt.

4.In a bowl add all the other ingredients.

5.Boil the mixture.

6.Let everything cool down.

7.Mix well and keep the mixture on the kitchen counter for 2-3 days.

Sauerkraut

Ingredients

1.Cabbage(450gm)

2.White salt (2 tbsp)

3.Pink salt (1 tbsp)

Method

1.Take 450 grams of cabbage.

2.Add white and pink salts.
3.Mix the ingredients well and firmly with your hands.
4.Leave for 30 minutes.
5.Add a little bit more salt water.
6.Put the ingredients in a glass jar.
7.Seal tightly after covering.
8.Leave for 3-5 days in the kitchen.
9.This is best consumed with rice or porridge.

CHAPTER VII

QUICK REVISION

#Plan your grocery items for a week.

#Switch to homemade drinks and snacks.

#Make your food interesting to make this change sustainable.

#Try to make your food nutrient-dense(mothers strategy).
#Hydrate your body with flavors and quality water.

#Chew your food properly.

#Don't just put water inside, drink it properly so that it actually quenches your thirst(sitting position)

#Take a sunbath every morning.

#Start your day with alkaline foods.

#Include oil pulling in your daily regime.

#Include infusion tea instead of "chai".

#Introduce fasting in your life.

#Add variations in your workout regime.

#Be mindful about supplements, don't take anything blindly.

#Utensils play an important role when it comes to your health, don't take this for granted.

#Spend some time with nature(indeed)

#Trust your doctors but not blindly.

Don't make excuses for your health.

Some add ons to your new life(the better you)

#Eat before 7 PM for better and proper digestion of food.

#Meditate or deep breathe(left nostril technique) for 5-7 minutes before sleeping at night.

#Cook rice in an open vessel instead of the pressure cooker.

#Oil your belly button before sleeping(few drops), you can use oils like coconut oil, neem oil, mustard oil.

#Take proper sleep, it has incredible power to heal your body and is very important to optimize immunity.

#Take care of your gut health.

"A Healthy Outside Starts From The Inside."
(Robert Urich)

CHAPTER VIII

PLAN OF ACTION

I don't want you to just read the book and forget. It's worthwhile for you as well as me only if you will implement whatever you have read in this book in your life. Start with the "1% rule" (Tommy Baker's book). The idea of the 1% rule is "if you can just consistently and persistently be 1% better at what you do each day, over the course of a year or a decade you will make significant progress. Specifically: So how do you motivate and organize yourself to be better every day?"

1.Fall in love with the process.
2.Do it every single day.
3.Celebrate your commitment.
4.Track your data

Fill this evaluation and check your progress every week:

Kindly rate these statements on a scale from 0 to 10	Start	Week 1	Week 2	Week 3	Week 4
How were your energy levels throughout the week?					
Waking up fresh or lethargic?					
Rate how satisfied you feel with the quality of sleep?					
Rate your bloating, indigestion, constipation, acidity.					
Rate your sweet cravings post-meal?					
Rate your satisfaction level after the workout.					
Rate your stress management.					
How satisfied are you with your water intake daily?					
Rate how satisfied you feel with sunbathing.					
How satisfied are you with your relations?					

CHAPTER IX

REFERENCES

https://www.aviyoggroup.in/

https://amerisleep.com/blog/

https://www.ncbi.nlm.nih.gov/

https://www.ncbi.nlm.nih.gov/pmc/articles/PMC1361287/#
https://pubmed.ncbi.nlm.nih.gov/

https://my.clevelandclinic.org/?_ga=2.175764459.811416437.1627411256136265994 0.1622805113&_gl=1*8m23ig*_ga*MTM2MjY1OTk0MC4xNjIyODA1MTEz*_ga_HWJ092SPKP*MTYyNzQxMTI1Ni4xMC4wLjE2Mjc0MTEyNTYuMA..

https://www.sunshineclinic.org/

https://medlineplus.gov/medlineplus.html
https://www.health.harvard.edu/

https://www.health.com/best-life-now

https://www.mayoclinic.org/

https://timesofindia.indiatimes.com/etimes

http://www.chemistry.wustl.edu/~edudev/LabTutorials/HIV/images/Immune.jpg

https://www.technologynetworks.com/

https://primaryimmune.org/

https://behealthyinstitute.com/

https://www.tcimedicine.com/

https://www.health.harvard.edu/

https://www.semanticscholar.org/https://doi.org/10.1016/J.JAUT.2007.07.014

https://silvermagazine.ca/

https://liveyourpassion.in/home

Dr.Tom O' Bryan, DC, CNN, DACBN, The dr.com, Faculty-institute of functional medicine, Chief health officer at knoWEwel

Jenna macchiochi Ph.D

Lecturer in Immunology(University of Sussex):: Contributing media Immunologist

https://www.mdpi.com

1.VP Research Institute, 287, Carlos Petit St, São Paulo 04110-000, Brazil

2.Department of Food Science and Technology, Federal University of Santa Maria, Rio Grande do Sul 97105-900, Brazil Author to whom correspondence should be addressed.

Nutrients **2017**, *9*(6), 538; https://doi.org/10.3390/nu9060538

Received: 27 March 2017 / Revised: 5 May 2017 / Accepted: 17 May 2017 / Published: 25 May 2017

https://www.health.harvard.edu/

https://www.nia.nih.gov/

https://www.webmd.com/fitness-exercise/default.htm

Michael Greger, M.D. FACLM, FOUNDER, NutritionFacts.org, Author-"How not to die"

www.ingramcontent.com/pod-product-compliance
Ingram Content Group UK Ltd.
Pitfield, Milton Keynes, MK11 3LW, UK
UKHW040032200726
13854UKWH00001B/485